CONSUMER GUIDE TO LONG-TERM CARE ■

Consumer Guide
to Long-Term Care

Gary R. Ilminen

THE UNIVERSITY OF WISCONSIN PRESS

The University of Wisconsin Press
2537 Daniels Street
Madison, Wisconsin 53718

3 Henrietta Street
London WC2E 8LU, England

5   4   3   2   1

Printed in the United States of America

Library of Congress Cataloging-in-Publication Data
Ilminen, Gary.
    Consumer guide to long-term care / by Gary Ilminen.
     256 pp.   cm.
     ISBN 0-299-16420-9 (cloth: alk. paper)
     ISBN 0-299-16424-1 (pbk.: alk. paper)
     1. Long-term care facilities—Utilization.   2. Aged—Long-term
  care.   3. Long-term care of the sick.   4. Consumer education.
    I. Title.
RA997.I46   1999
362.1'6—dc21   99-14422

For my parents, Roy and Elaine Ilminen,
and millions of moms and dads
all over the country just like them
who deserve the best we can give them

And for my children, Jesse, Brady, and Elaina

CONTENTS ■

FIGURES ■

TABLES ■

ACKNOWLEDGMENTS ■

It is difficult to do justice to all the people who have contributed to the creation of this book. That multitude includes hundreds of individuals whose care needs brought their lives into contact with mine, thus making mine the richer. Their interesting lives, their often surprising and remarkable stories, their humor, compassion, and wisdom taught me a great deal. Through them, I learned the true value of the work done by all the people employed in nursing homes and, indeed, in all health care settings. Thus my first acknowledgment is to those remarkable people whom I had the opportunity to care for over the years; they gave me a great deal, even though they probably did not realize it. It is for them, their families, and millions like them that I felt this book was necessary. They are the ones who gave me purpose throughout this book's creation, which has spanned several years.

Next, the many colleagues I have enjoyed working with in my nursing career have given me encouragement and advice and challenged my thinking as this book took shape. Most helped in the development of my knowledge base over the years. Fellow RNs, LPNs, nursing assistants, pharmacists, physicians, physician's assistants, state surveyors, administrators, dieticians, housekeeping, maintenance, activities, and social services staff members I have worked with and met in the course of my work have all contributed from their own experience. They possess a remarkably specialized set of skills that most people do not develop an appreciation for. I am fortunate to have worked with individuals in these areas, who have taught me a great deal over the years.

I wish to give special thanks to the highly skilled professionals who offered their time and expertise in providing critical review of the manuscript. Gerald C. Kempthorne, MD, I thank with particular recognition for his thoughtful insights and suggestions on the manuscript. Dr. Kempthorne is a widely recognized practitioner in southern Wisconsin with more than thirty years of long-term care experience, including work as a nursing home medical director. His support and suggestions enlivened this project.

Special thanks to Judith C. Fryback, director, Bureau of Quality Assurance, and Dinh Tran, health services consultant, each with the State of Wisconsin, Department of Health and Family Services, Madison, for their technical review. Their insights on the technical aspects of the manuscript with respect to the survey requirements, MDS information, and long-term care facility certification requirements were of enormous help.

Thanks to Bruce A. Kraus, MD, for his support and insightful review of the manuscript. Dr. Kraus is president of Cornucopian Health Concepts of Columbus, Wisconsin; he is a family practice primary care physician and medical director for two skilled-nursing facilities. He is also past president of the Wisconsin Nursing Home Medical Director's Association. His review based on his long experience in health care was extremely helpful in development of the manuscript.

Thanks also to Pamela M. Mokler, whose experience in gerontology and managed care and experience as a long-term care ombudsman formed the basis for excellent observations on the structure and content of the manuscript. Ms. Mokler received her master of science degree in gerontology from California State University and is co-founder of Quality Aging Solutions of Costa Mesa, California.

Thanks to E. Jane Danielson for her thoughtful review of the manuscript and support for the project. Ms. Danielson is a freelance writer with firsthand knowledge of long-term care for a loved one from a consumer's perspective.

Particular thanks to the editorial committee and to the professional staff of the University of Wisconsin Press: Dr. Rosalie M. Robertson, senior acquisitions editor for the press, who recognized the importance of this project and helped move it forward; Scott Lenz, senior editor, whose patience and expertise helped guide this project to successful completion; Kris Coppens, acquisition assistant, whose professional attitude and encouragement greatly assisted me in the earliest stages of publication. Thanks to the many other staff at the University of Wisconsin Press who contributed to the publication of *Consumer Guide to Long-Term Care.* Special thanks to Carole Schwager for her excellent copyediting of the manuscript.

Gary R. Ilminen
Prairie du Sac, Wisconsin
May 1999

There are more than 1.66 million nursing home beds available in the United States in more than 16,700 nursing homes across the country. These facilities provide essential long-term health care services for the chronically ill individual as well as short-term convalescent care, yet entry into the system can be an extremely stressful event for recipients of the care as well as their spouses and families.

Whether the decision to place a loved one in a long-term care facility is compelled by a gradual deterioration of some physical condition to a point where spouse or family members can no longer meet the individual's needs or by a sudden event such as a stroke or injury, it imposes huge changes on the individual and the family and does so in a very short time. About 68 percent of people admitted to nursing homes are admitted directly from acute care hospitals.[1] This generally means that time to study nursing homes to determine the best choice and time to prepare for a long-term care stay will be limited.

Consequently, not only are individuals who need care burdened with concerns about their own health status, but they must often make myriad decisions and answer hundreds of questions that they simply were not prepared to deal with. In many cases, if the patient cannot do these things for medical reasons, such as a dementing illness or severe memory loss, the spouse or the family must handle these issues. This compounds the stress of dealing with a loved one's illness and can lead to strong disagreements among family members, confusion over the many forms and consents that must be signed, fears of the financial consequences of the illness, and even stress-related health problems for those thrust unexpectedly into this process.

Complicating this process is the rapid change taking place in the nursing home business. Consumers increasingly find themselves dealing not with the locally owned "mom-and-pop" nursing home of the past but with corporate giants that generate hundreds of millions of dollars in annual revenue, operate nationwide, and have slick, sophisticated management systems and policies. When policies that affect how the facility is operated are made at some distant corporate headquarters, consumers and families raising quality-of-care, quality-of-life, and residents' rights issues may have difficulty ensuring their voices are heard.

1. *Hoechst Marion Roussel Institutional Digest 1996.*

The funding systems for long-term care are also going through major changes and growing increasingly complex. The Medicare program is changing how it pays nursing homes and home health agencies for the care they provide, moving them to a prospective payment system. This system will result in per-day payments to nursing facilities that are adjusted for the complexity of the facility's case mix. Based on a set of adjustment factors called resource utilization groups (RUGs) developed in a project called the Nursing Home Case Mix and Quality Demonstration project, the system sets the rate of reimbursement to the facility per day (per diem) based on how much care residents require.

More and more people who are eligible for Medicare are entering health maintenance organizations (HMOs). The Balanced Budget Act of 1997 will have the effect of moving more people into some form of managed care. Offering a dizzying alphabet soup of managed care options, the Medicare+Choice provisions of the law are intended to give Medicare beneficiaries more options for access to their Medicare benefits. But managed care imposes limits and rules, and it can cause confusion for consumers as well.

People eligible for coverage under the Medicaid (Medical Assistance) program face changes in that system as well. By 1998, at least 49 states moved much of their Medicaid population into HMOs. Most of the recipients affected are younger individuals with young children in their families. Also, by 1998, nine states were expanding the use of Medicaid managed care to include elderly individuals and those with physical and developmental disabilities. These systems may affect both quality of care and length of stay for people using nursing homes.

The goal of this guide is to provide a comprehensive resource for consumers who suddenly find themselves facing the need for placement in a long-term care facility or who must cope with the placement of a loved one. I hope to help prevent the stresses associated with such placement by outlining what to look for in preplanning long-term care placement whenever that can be done; by offering ready reference materials designed to help explain the myriad laws and rules affecting everything from admission to discharge, resident rights, quality of care, costs, who pays and how; and by providing a comprehensive listing of additional resources and agencies available to help you.

Consumer Guide to Long-Term Care goes beyond providing information about how to select a nursing home and explaining how public and private payer sources work. This book is designed to empower consumers and their families to have a meaningful influence over the quality of care and quality of life experienced in the nursing home at the level of the individual as well as facilitywide. It is written to give consumers the information they need to evaluate the quality of the services provided by a nursing home, to recognize critical problems that degrade quality of life for nursing home residents, including some that are subtle or technical in nature, and to be effective advocates for quality improvement.

Consumer Guide to Long-Term Care is also designed to inform consumers about how to get the latest performance information concerning quality-of-care issues on any nursing home in the country, and how well the regulatory system that governs nursing homes is working. This book seeks to replace fear and distrust of nursing homes with knowledge and a feeling of empowerment that will allow consumers to work with nursing homes in order to prevent and resolve problems and thereby to ensure loved ones will experience the highest quality of life possible in a long-term care facility.

HOW TO USE THIS GUIDE ■

The best and most advantageous way for you to use this guide depends on your circumstances. If you are in the fortunate position to be doing some advance planning and the need to arrange long-term care is not a pressing situation, you can select the topics you wish to explore at your leisure. In that case, going chapter by chapter from front to back will work nicely.

If you need to arrange long-term care or rehabilitation in a short time frame, you may wish to go straight to chapter 5 "Choosing a Long-Term Care Facility." If that chapter makes you wonder how to pay for care, "Paying for Care" would be the next chapter to read. If you are still uncertain about the types of care and facilities out there and need to get a basic understanding of who does what, the first chapter, "Long-Term Care Defined," will be valuable. If you are dealing with an HMO for coverage of the care, either under a "commercial" line of insurance from your employer or under a Medicare HMO or Medicaid HMO product, chapter 3, "HMOs," will be useful.

If you are already a recipient of care in a facility or are the decision maker, advocate, guardian, or family member for someone who is, then simply select the topic of most immediate interest to you. For example, if your loved one has been diagnosed with Alzheimer's disease and you have questions about the disease and the care that can be given, the chapter on Alzheimer's disease should be of help. Other topics in that circumstance may arise as well, for example, the use of psychoactive medications and physical restraints. Read "Powerful Stuff: Rules That Protect You from the Misuse of Psychoactive Medications" and "Don't Tie Me Down! The Right to Be Free from the Use of Physical Restraints" for help with these difficult and often controversial topics.

If you are involved in care planning or want to review the medical record (chart), you should find appendix A, "Common Health Care Acronyms and Abbreviations," at the back of the book to be useful. Care planning begins at the point of admission to the facility and usually includes discussion about advance directives. In that case, chapters 8 and 9 deal with the medical record and chapters 11, 15, 16, 17, and 18 deal with various aspects of your advance directive.

Throughout the text, I define terms and acronyms in parentheses when they are first used. If you encounter an unfamiliar term or abbreviation with no accompanying definition, check in appendix A. Throughout the text, I try to make a lot of technical and sometimes complex jargon understandable and useful by writing in an informal and informative style. I not only tell you about the technical rules that affect your long-term care experience, but put them into context so you can see how they apply in the delivery of care.

In the text, I use the term "you" in a catchall way to refer to the reader—including the recipient of the care as well as the interested third party such as a guardian, advocate, attorney-in-fact, or family member. This should cause no confusion, but you will need to take this into consideration in applying the material to a given situation.

Finally, this text is intended to provide much-needed consumer protection information on long-term care. It is intended as a guide to help you prepare for a long-term care experience, to raise it to the highest level of satisfaction and effectiveness, and to help you develop expectations of your caregivers that are both high and realistic. Use this guide as a tool to help you deal with caregivers, facility management, and insurers as an informed consumer. Use it *not* as a substitute for the assistance of appropriate agencies, competent legal advice, or the skill of your physician but, rather, as a resource to help you know where and when to get such assistance.

In my opinion, there is no foolproof way to identify a "good" or "bad" nursing home. My belief is that any nursing home, on any given day, is capable of providing good, compassionate care or substandard, negligent care. The fact is, your ability to identify which facilities have the track record and organization and staffing to *enable* them to do a good job is a good start on the road to a satisfying episode of care. This book provides the tools to do that. Informed consumers who have the ability to identify key quality-of-care issues and who can recognize high quality of care and demand it of facilities can do far more to improve the industry than any army of state survey (inspection) teams ever could. Consumers can be in the facilities every day, if they feel the need. Survey teams simply can't.

The goal of this book is to help consumers learn what "quality of care" means and get it for themselves or their loved ones in every facility, for every day of care, in every area of their lives in long-term care.

1

Long-Term Care Defined

In health care, the phrase "continuum of care" is often used to refer to the utilization of the full range of necessary health services required to restore an individual's health. The continuum of care allows the level of care services to match the health care needs of the individual—ideally allowing the individual to get the care needed for the length of time required in the appropriate setting and for the least cost to the consumer.

In the United States, the continuum of care is defined as much by the kind of facility as by the nature of the services provided. In general, the following definitions apply.

■

HOSPITAL CARE

ACUTE CARE

Care provided by hospitals, often for sudden illnesses or injuries expected to last only a short time. The government pays for care provided to individuals through Medicare by a system called **prospective payment:** a fixed dollar amount based on the main or primary admitting diagnosis, known as a diagnosis-related group (DRG), which uses the average length of a hospital stay for the main diagnosis, is the basis for payment. This system ignores the length of the hospital stay and even the actual cost of providing the care. The goal is cost containment and the approach is being used more and more by private insurers as well. Hospitals have been profoundly affected: literally hundreds of small, rural hospitals have been closed and many elderly patients are discharged from the hospital while still quite ill, leading many in the health care profession to say that patients are being discharged from the hospital "quicker and sicker." It has also led to more frequent use of long-term care facilities as the destination after hospital discharge, since patients are often in need of care that cannot be provided at home, even with home health services.

NURSING HOME CARE

SUBACUTE CARE

Complex medical care for serious or multiple medical conditions that are likely to last a long time. Individuals requiring subacute care may be placed in one of a growing number of facilities, which may be individual facilities or part of a nursing home, and some are actually a part of an acute care hospital. An individual receiving long-term life support on a ventilator is an example of someone receiving subacute care.

NURSING FACILITY (NF)

Facility offering long-term health care, formerly called nursing home or rest home. Today, nursing facilities generally are certified for Medicaid, but not for payment under Medicare. The term "skilled nursing facility" refers to a nursing home certified for the Medicare program. Many skilled nursing facilities are certified for both programs or are considered "dually certified." Medicare generally does not reimburse for NF care.

SKILLED NURSING FACILITY (SNF)

Facility that provides complex medical and nursing care as well as a variety of other therapeutic specialties such as physical therapy, occupational therapy, speech therapy, and respiratory therapy. The full range of basic care services that a person may need—such as assistance with bathing, dressing, mobility, and personal hygiene—is provided. In addition, SNFs offer specialized treatments such as intravenous fluids, parenteral nutrition (giving life-sustaining nutrients by an intravenous route), and enteral nutrition (giving nutrition by the use of a tube into the stomach). Medicare pays for many of the services provided in a skilled nursing facility, but only for a limited time.

INTERMEDIATE CARE FACILITY (ICF)

Facility offering care that focuses on chronic but relatively less complex conditions that may require supervision and observation, not constant intervention. This type of care is often referred to as "custodial care." Nursing services include medication administration, injections, wound care, nutritional therapy that does not require the use of intravenous or feeding tubes, skin care, and assistance with activities of daily living (ADLs) such as bathing, dressing, grooming, toileting, mobility, and personal hygiene. Medicare, in general, does not reimburse for ICF care, but Medicaid may pay for much of the care needed for individuals who meet eligibility criteria. The ICF type of facility is no longer recognized in federal regulations, but the designation continues to be used in some states.

ASSISTED LIVING CENTERS

Facility offering some degree of assistance with personal care as well as providing laundry and housekeeping services. They usually are not licensed to provide nursing care but may have a system that makes a nurse available to residents for assistance with medications or in the case of illness. Assisted living centers are not reimbursed by Medicare and 20 states will cover assisted living under Medicaid, but usually they must be paid directly by the consumer. Some states may have board-and-care facilities that function like assisted living; seven states cover board-and-care under Medicaid.

HOME HEALTH SERVICES

In-home provision of skilled nursing services, a variety of therapies such as physical, speech, occupational, and respiratory therapy, assistance with ADLs such as bathing, dressing, hygiene, and other personal care. These services can initially be paid for by Medicare and when that runs out by state Medicaid funding, if the individual qualifies. Other state and local funding sources exist in some localities. A key difference between home health care and care in the nursing facility is that the individual must be able to function safely at home or have live-in help for much of the time.

GETTING TO KNOW THE NURSING HOME (AND WHY THAT IS IMPORTANT)

No two nursing homes are exactly alike. As hard as both the regulators and corporate owners may have tried to reduce the industry to one common, cookie-cutter formula for the ideal, it just has not happened, and it will not happen. The business of providing hands-on long-term care is a distinctly human enterprise—and one that defies codification and standardization in many areas. That is why I have come to the conclusion that there is no intrinsically "good" or "bad" nursing home.

Every facility has the potential to do a great job on a given case on any given day. Likewise, every facility has the potential to do a lousy job on a given case on a given day. It is because of this tendency toward wide variations that I wrote this book. The difference between the good and bad, for consumers can be as narrow as one bad incident, one staff member having a bad day, or one bad staff member. Worse, it must be said that there are some facilities out there that are badly managed, chronically short-staffed, poorly maintained, and very unlikely to be able to deliver the quality of care and quality of life their residents deserve.

Informed consumers can help tip the scales in favor of quality care because they can be there more often than regulators and can advocate more effectively at the local level. Working with a nursing home to lobby for quality care, quality of life, and residents' rights can be time-consuming and frustrating, especially if you do not understand how nursing homes operate, do not know the rules, or cannot speak the language. The bulk of this book addresses the two latter issues. In this section, you will get to know a little about how nursing homes operate.

ORGANIZATION, ADMINISTRATION, AND INFORMATION

The days of the locally owned, mom-and-pop nursing home appear to be ending. As figure 1 illustrates, between 1985 and 1995 ownership of nursing homes shifted from individuals to corporate chains. This is neither necessarily bad nor good; it is simply a fact. What this fact may mean to

consumers, though, is that no matter where the nursing home you are dealing with gets its marching orders from, the rules discussed in this book apply. However, the interpretation and implementation of the policies the corporate hierarchy may create can have an effect on quality of care and quality of life for the people in their care. If the distant corporate headquarters is difficult to communicate with and the local administration is unresponsive to consumers' issues, problems may be corrected at a snail's pace—or not at all.

To prevent this, it is helpful to know how the nursing home you are dealing with is structured and who the decision makers are. Start with the layer of the organization closest to the resident—the direct care staff. This will include the nursing assistants, restorative aides, activity aides, the licensed practical nurses (LPNs), the registered nurses (RNs), dietary staff, maintenance, housekeeping and laundry staff, and so on. Talk first to the people who are closest to the issue. They often are the ones who will be called on to solve the problem anyway, and often they can make changes that are effective immediately.

Of course, if a member of the staff *is* the problem, you may need to take the issue to the first level of supervision or to the social services department (see chapter 14). Some problems, though, are of a systemwide nature. These will usually need to be dealt with from some level of the administration. The "typical" nursing facility will have an organizational structure that divides various responsibilities among groups or departments. There are, of course, a multitude of variations on this structure; some facilities will have more, others less.

The facility must have a *governing body,* to whom the entire organization within the facility is ultimately responsible. For county-owned or tribal facilities, this may be the county board, the tribal council, the county social services board, or another body designated by the county or tribe. For privately owned facilities, it may be a corporate board of directors or a board convened by the corporation and designated to act as the governing body. The governing body has final responsibility for the policies and operation of the facility and for appointment of a qualified administrator. Consumers should find out who is on a facility's governing

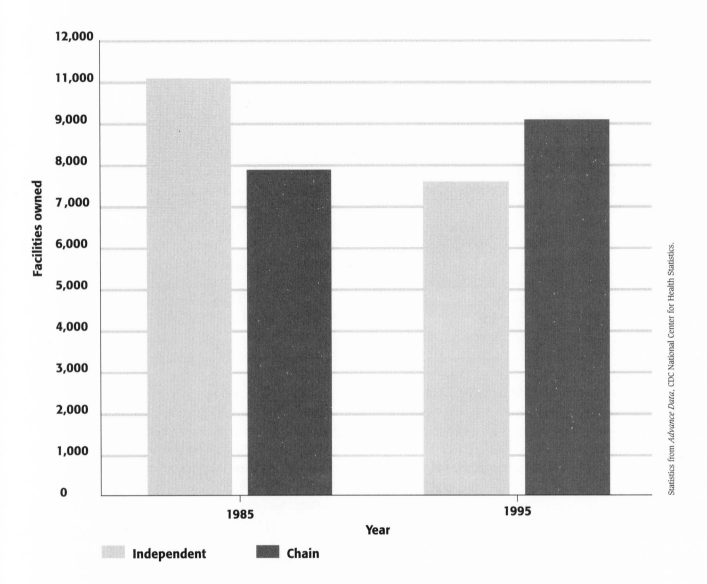

Statistics from *Advance Data*, CDC National Center for Health Statistics.

Ownership of nursing homes is changing, with "mom and pop" nursing homes disappearing as chains take over the industry. In 1985, some 11,100 (58.1 percent) of the nation's nursing homes were independently owned and 7,900 (41.3 percent) of the homes were controlled by corporate chains. By 1995, big chains had gobbled up thousands of independents to control 9,100 (54.4 percent of the industry) while independently owned facilities declined to 7,600 homes (45.5 percent of the industry). For consumers, this means talking to "the owner" of the facility about problems is less likely to be possible. Does it necessarily mean poor quality? That depends in large part on the corporation.

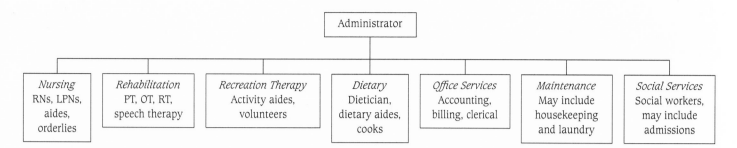

			Administrator			
Nursing RNs, LPNs, aides, orderlies	*Rehabilitation* PT, OT, RT, speech therapy	*Recreation Therapy* Activity aides, volunteers	*Dietary* Dietician, dietary aides, cooks	*Office Services* Accounting, billing, clerical	*Maintenance* May include housekeeping and laundry	*Social Services* Social workers, may include admissions

body and how to reach them; this information can be useful if issues taken to the level of the administrator do not seem to be getting resolved, though that step should rarely be necessary.

Facility administration requires a versatile, resilient individual with a variety of technical, management, and "people" skills. Within the facility, the administrator is responsible for all aspects of the operation. The rules governing nursing home operations[1] state that each facility must be administered in a manner that

> *enables it to use its resources effectively and efficiently to attain or maintain the highest practicable physical, mental and psychosocial well-being of each resident.*
>
> *[42 CFR Sec. 483.75]*

This short statement is a tall order. Compliance with the rules discussed in this book is a difficult and vital job. It has been said that the rules for operating a nursing home are more numerous and complicated than those for operating a nuclear power plant; this may not be far from true. Even if it is true, it does not excuse poor facility performance, but it does give the reader a perspective on how tough the job is to do well.

There are, in fact, a great many administrators who run excellent facilities. They talk to consumers, families, their staff, and the community. They listen and respond to what they hear. Some find imaginative ways to enhance the quality of life for the people in their care and for the people who render the care. They lead by example and find the time to go beyond budget headaches and paperwork compliance issues to be advocates for the *people* who call the facility home. They make decisions based on what is best for residents and expect the same from their staff.

Leaders in long-term care are swamped with regulations. They will agree that a certain amount of documentation must be created to manage and improve quality of care, but the greater the burden of paperwork becomes, the less time is available for providing care and designing imaginative solutions to quality problems. Though each department in a nursing home has a share of responsibility for paperwork as well as the delivery of services, some of the most complicated and important falls within the nursing department.

NURSING SERVICES

Many of the key quality-of-care, quality-of-life, and residents' rights responsibilities associated with nursing home care are directly linked to the daily activities of the nursing department in the facility. These issues and their relation to various operations of the facility are dealt with individually later in the book; here we consider nursing services in general terms.

The greatest share of a nursing facility's labor budget typically is spent on the nursing staff. In sheer numbers, the

---

1. All rules that appear in boxes are from the *State Operations Manual: Provider Certification,* Guidance to Surveyors—Long-Term Care Facilities, HCFA, July 1995. They can be found in the *Code of Federal Regulations* (CFR), at the sections cited.

nursing staff is the largest group of employees in virtually all facilities. This staff includes the director of nursing, assistant director of nursing (if any), nurse managers, unit managers, care coordinators, medication or special treatment nurses, a variety of other nurse specialists that the facility may have, shift supervisors, staff nurses, and the nursing assistants (see also chapter 12).

Large staff size, numerous hours of contact, and diversity of services provided through nursing in a facility add up to a major impact on the experience of care for a facility's residents and their families. Consequently, a great deal of regulation of the who, what, when, where, and why of care focuses on services provided by the nursing staff. As a result, a great deal of the documentation load also falls on the nursing department. This causes a lot of nursing time to be spent focused on "paper compliance"—documentation created to meet regulatory requirements. There is a growing sentiment among advocates and regulators alike that consumers would be better served if the focus were shifted away from paper compliance toward actual *outcomes* of care. While that holds promise, it may lead to yet more paperwork as regulators construct data gathering requirements to measure outcomes, while not relieving any of the current paperwork requirements.

The nursing staff must be adequate to meet the needs of the residents living in the facility. That requirement is stated in the rules for nursing homes this way:

> *The facility must have sufficient nursing staff to provide nursing and related services to attain or maintain the highest practicable physical, mental, and psychosocial well-being of each resident, and as determined by resident assessments, and individual plans of care.*
>
> *[42 CFR Sec. 483.30]*

Ask most nursing assistants and they will tell you that being "short-staffed" is one of their most common problems. The same could be said for the RN and LPN staff. Finding (and keeping) enough skilled and dedicated people to do

this difficult work is an ongoing struggle in the long-term care industry. When the facility is understaffed, the staff that *are* present must work at a feverish pace, leaving them fatigued, frazzled, and frustrated. The residents can often sense this happening, and it may be abundantly clear in the quality of care, staff attitude, and time it takes to get a response to the call light.

The nursing staff requirements include both nursing assistants and licensed nurses (RNs, LPNs, etc.). The facility must have licensed nursing staff present 24 hours a day, unless the facility has been granted a waiver of the requirement by the state. It also must have an RN present at least eight hours a day, seven days a week, unless granted a waiver by the state. The facility must also designate a licensed nurse to act as a charge nurse on each shift, unless it has been granted a waiver for this requirement. Finally, the facility must designate an RN to serve as a director of nursing on a full-time basis. The duties of director of nursing may be shared by two RNs, but their hours in that capacity must total 40 hours per week and each must understand the responsibilities of the job.

■
GETTING TO KNOW THE PROVIDERS

It's useful to know who does what in the long-term care setting and what some of those initials you may see after caregivers' names mean.

AD

The *activity director* plans and carries out diversional activities, or recreation therapy, for residents. Such activities are required at nursing facilities; they may include group activities like van outings, parties, and movies as well as individualized activities of interest to each resident.

LPN

The *licensed practical nurse,* typically a graduate of a one-year course of study, may occupy the role of charge nurse, give medications, do certain dressing changes, and make physical assessments. The LPN is known in some jurisdictions as an **LVN,** or *licensed vocational nurse.*

MD/DO

The *doctor of medicine* or *doctor of osteopathy* is the individual with crucial case management responsibility, issuing medical orders for care and treatment. In most jurisdictions, a psychiatrist must also be an MD. In the long-term care facility setting, the MD or DO who is the *attending physician* is required to do regular evaluations of his or her patients and should do at least every other hands-on assessment personally. The MD or DO will give orders for day-to-day care for the nursing staff and other clinical specialists to follow (see chapter 11).

NA

The *nursing assistant* or *nurse's aide* is a key figure in the provision of bedside care—bathing, dressing, hygiene, grooming, range of motion exercises, skin care, and the like. You may also see **CNA** for *certified nursing assistant,* **CENA** for *competency-evaluated nursing assistant,* or **NA-R,** meaning *nursing assistant–registered.* The term "nursing assistant" is sometimes used to refer to an individual who, because of length of service, is not required to pass the clinical and written tests required under new federal laws to prove competency as a caregiver. The other titles generally apply only to those who have taken and passed the competency tests (see chapter 12).

NHA

The *nursing home administrator* must generally be licensed by the state, usually based on the completion of a specialized course of study or program. Administrators can have a variety of backgrounds by education and experience. Many have degrees in social work, nursing, business administration, or a combination of these and others. An administrator with a strong resident/family focus is a major factor in nursing home quality.

OT

The *occupational therapist* works to increase or maintain function and mobility in the smaller muscle groups of the arms and hands. Goals of the OT typically include restoration of manual skills for eating, writing, and dressing and may include teaching the individual how to do these things using adaptive devices. Preparation requires a bachelor's degree and additional clinical training. **COTA** stands for *certified occupational therapy assistant.*

PA-C

The *physician's assistant–certified* typically has a baccalaureate degree and additional training in medicine and biology, but has not completed medical school. The PA-C has prescribing authority under physician supervision. A state certification or licensing exam is required.

PhD

A clinician or psychologist will generally hold a *doctor of philosophy* degree.

PT

The goals of the *physical therapist* are to increase or preserve function, strength, and mobility in the limbs and large muscle groups. Physical therapists may have a two- or four-year degree, and most states require licensure.

RD

A *registered dietician* develops diet plans and menus to meet each resident's nutritional needs in compliance with the doctor's orders. Generally the RD will also supervise the staff of the dietary department in the preparation of meals. Dieticians may be registered by the Commission on Dietetic Registration of the American Dietetic Association or qualified based on state requirements.

RN

A *registered nurse* can be licensed to practice with this title after two years of college in an associate degree program, three years in what is known as a diploma program, or four years in a bachelor's degree program (BSN). An RN who holds a master's degree in nursing (MSN) and other qualifications depending on the licensing requirements may practice as a *nurse clinician* or *nurse practitioner.* In some cases, these advanced-practice nurses may write prescriptions and orders as a physician would. In the long-term care setting, RN staff are generally in the charge nurse role, do skilled assessments, start intravenous drips, place nasogastric tubes, administer medications, change dressings, perform other skilled care procedures, and conduct observation. Nurses occupy a number of administrative roles, such as director of nursing (DON), resident services managers, and clinical care coordinators.

RPh

The *registered pharmacist* reviews each patient's medication regime at regular intervals to ensure that each medication is given for an appropriate diagnosis, in the lowest effective dose, and for the shortest period of time. As a result of recent changes in the law, the nursing facility's consultant pharmacist is a key figure in the management of each resident's care from the standpoint of the medications that he or she receives. The pharmacist must also look for potential drug interactions, be aware of allergies, and be alert for possible medication errors in transcription of orders or administration (see chapter 19).

ST

As the name suggests, the *speech therapist* will focus on restoration of the individual's ability to speak, which may have been affected by a stroke or surgery. He or she also fulfills a vital role in working with patients with dysphagia (difficulty swallowing). A *speech-language pathologist,* or **SLP,** may also be involved in identifying and treating problems with chewing, swallowing, or speaking.

SW

The duties and qualifications of the *social worker* may vary from one jurisdiction or facility to another, but the key func-

tions generally revolve around organizing personal and financial data on each resident, assisting with financial resources or problems, identifying and helping to resolve resident personal, social, psychosocial, emotional, and mental problems, and helping with the adjustment to life in the facility.

There are other caregivers, of course but these are the individuals who nursing facility residents and their families come in contact with most frequently. There is, however, one more acronym that has had profound impact on the nursing home business that we need to cover as we define long-term care—**OBRA.**

■

WHAT IS OBRA?

No, OBRA is not the name of a talk-show host. It is the abbreviated name of the Omnibus Budget Reconciliation Act of 1987, federal legislation regulating how nursing homes in this country do business. The OBRA legislation includes the most comprehensive nursing home reform package ever written. The rules are officially known as the Medicare and Medicaid Long-Term Care Facility Requirements.

Springing from the work of consumer advocacy groups such as the National Citizens' Coalition for Nursing Home Reform (NCCNHR) and research by the Institute of Medicine,[2] the rules in OBRA were designed to address many problems, some very serious, in the long-term care industry. The rules specifically apply to any nursing home that receives Medicare or Medicaid dollars and is dependent on certification for continued operation. However, the rules have become the model for quality standards that have been developed for use on non–Medicare- or Medicaid-certified facilities as well.

Sweeping in scope, the legislation affects almost every aspect of long-term care, but it is particularly emphatic on the subjects of quality of life, quality of care, residents' rights,

---

2. The IOM is a component of the National Academy of Sciences. Chartered in 1970, the IOM enlists top members of various professions to examine policy matters pertaining to public health.

admission, discharge and transfer rights, resident behavior and facility practices, resident assessment, and physical environment.

A good portion of this book is designed to inform you of the rights and protections provided by this landmark legislation, what the law says and what it means in terms of the care provided, and how to ensure that those rights and requirements are upheld.

2

Paying for Care

Short of the concerns generated by the health conditions that lead to the need for long-term care in the first place, perhaps no issue is as burdensome as handling the financial impact of paying for care. Long-term care in a nursing home can be extremely expensive. According to the Health Insurance Association of America, the national average cost for a year of nursing home care can range from $36,000 to $60,000. The association also reports that the cost of having an aide deliver custodial care like bathing, dressing, and chore services in your own home only three times a week can cost $12,000 a year. Skilled therapy services can raise the cost significantly.

Fortunately, resources are available to help cover the cost of long-term care for many people, and these resources are discussed in this chapter. According to the Health Care Financing Administration (HCFA) Center for Information Systems, Medicaid paid for 68.4 percent of the long-term care delivered in nursing homes in the United States in 1995. Private payment by the consumer and private insurance accounted for 23.6 percent in 1995; Medicare covered about 8 percent of the cases (see figure 2). According to the *Hoechst Marion Roussel Institutional Digest 1996,* the Veterans Administration covered about 1.1 percent of the cases, and HMOs covered about 0.7 percent. Since Medicaid is such a significant source of payment, we look at it first.

■

MEDICAID (ALSO MEDICAL ASSISTANCE)

The Medicaid program originated at the federal level. Although it is funded by both state and federal sources, the program is administered by the states and rules and coverages can vary somewhat from state to state. You can obtain specific information on rules, eligibility requirements, and covered services from your state office of social services, state agency on aging, or state Medicaid office. See the resource directory at the back of this guide (appendix B) for more information.

Since the rules can vary from state to state, we consider Medicaid in general terms only. The first thing to know about Medicaid is that eligibility is based on economic resources—that is, it is not for everybody. Not everyone can qualify to receive payment for long-term care by Medicaid because the program is designed to pay for care for individuals with low income and limited

FIGURE 2: PAYER SOURCES IN LONG-TERM CARE, 1991–1995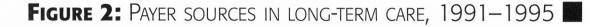

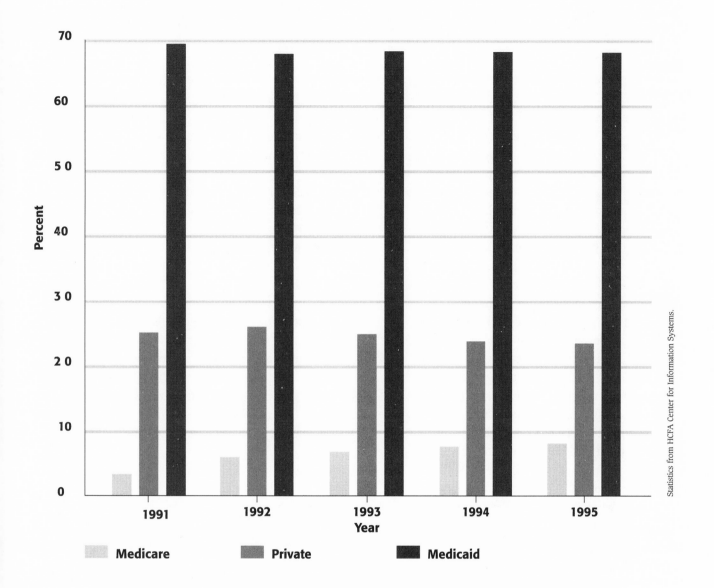

Statistics from HCFA Center for Information Systems.

Another effect of OBRA 1987 has been an increase in the number of long-term care residents admitted for care under the Medicare program. Although Medicaid still covered 68.4 percent of the long-term care in 1995, down slightly from 69.9 percent in 1991, the Medicaid program was still the dominant source of funding for long-term care. Medicare increased to 8 percent of the funding picture by 1995, up from 5.2 percent in 1991. This increase resulted partly from the increased number of beds certified for skilled nursing care under the Medicare program due to the significantly higher reimbursement under Medicare compared to Medicaid. Private insurance paid for 25.2 percent of care in 1991 and actually decreased slightly to 23.6 percent by 1995.

financial assets. The qualifying limits of financial assets vary by state. You will need to work with your local social services department or the social worker at the facility where admission is to occur to find out if you qualify for Medicaid coverage.

It is important to remember that even if you cannot qualify for Medicaid at the time of admission to a facility, it is possible to "spend down" to the qualifying level of financial assets and then become eligible for coverage. "Spend down" refers to paying for care on your own until your assets decrease to the level allowing qualification for Medicaid. It may be necessary to reapply for Medicaid at that time, so contact your local social services office when you believe you qualify. Again, the social worker at the facility providing care can help you with this process.

At one time, the qualifying limits for Medicaid were so low that the spouse remaining at home faced living in poverty. Recent changes in the law, however, have set higher limits on retained assets and income so the spend-down period can be shorter and the financial implications for the spouse at home not as bleak. In general, Medicaid will continue to pay for covered services as long as the care is necessary and the individual continues to meet the qualification requirements. However, if the person's financial assets or income increases, say, due to an inheritance or sale of property, the individual may temporarily become ineligible if the change exceeds the asset or income level allowed. Such changes must be reported to the social services office administering Medicaid benefits in your area.

Once the financial eligibility requirements are met, Medicaid will cover a significant number of the goods and services necessary for care in a nursing home, including what is known as **custodial care**: assistance with walking, bathing, dressing, eating, grooming, hygiene, taking medications, and the like. This is important since this is the kind of care that most nursing facility residents require but Medicare does *not* cover.

The following list of supplies and services provided is not complete or inclusive for all states or circumstances but indicates items generally covered by Medicaid for a nursing facility resident. Some states may include more, others less, and still other things can be covered in certain cases when medically necessary (ordered by your physician) and given prior authorization by the state Medicaid office.

MEDICAL/NURSING SERVICES

administration of medications

application of protective restraints, orthotics, prostheses, or postural device

bed baths or assistance with bathing, dressing, and self-care

care plan development

cast care

chest percussion/postural drainage

continuous administration of IV fluids and/or oxygen

drawing blood samples and lab work

exercise, range of motion teaching, and assistance

feeding and nutrition planning

instruction for maintenance therapy

nasopharyngeal aspiration (suctioning the upper airway)

nebulizer treatments (for respiratory disorders)

ostomy and catheter care

patient positioning and decubitus care (to treat or prevent skin breakdown known as bedsores)

restorative nursing procedures

skilled nursing observation

skin care

tube feedings

vital signs monitoring

wound dressing changes

COMMON MEDICAL EQUIPMENT AND SUPPLIES

atomizers

bed, linens, and associated equipment

bedside stands

blood pressure equipment

canes, crutches, and walkers

catheters and associated supplies

chair cushions

commodes

cotton balls and swabs

deodorizers

diagnostic agents (test kits)

disposable gloves

dressings and bandaging materials

elastic hose (antiembolus stockings, also called TED [thromboembolic disease] hose)

emesis basins

enema kits

finger cots

first aid supplies

flameproof cubicle curtains

footboards

footstools

freestanding meal trays

geriatric chairs (often called "geri-chairs")

hot water bottles

hypodermic needles/syringes

ice bags

incontinency supplies including pads, briefs, and liners

infrared lamps

irrigation solutions

IV supplies and equipment

lifts (for patient self-assistance rising)

nebulizers

ostomy supplies

oxygen equipment and supplies

plastic waste bags

positioning pads and devices

reading lights

recreational/therapeutic equipment or supplies for diversional activities

sitz baths

splints and slings

suction machines

traction equipment for orthopedic care

trapeze equipment (for patient self-positioning)

thermometers

tongue blades

tracheostomy care supplies

trochanter rolls (devices used for patient positioning)

tublifts

urinals

washbasins

water carafes and glasses

wheelchairs

Personal Hygiene Items

bacteriostatic soap

body lotions

combs and brushes

deodorant

facial tissues

hair conditioners

medicine cups

oral hygiene supplies including toothbrushes, toothpaste and denture cleaners, and mouthwash

patient gowns

safety razors

sanitary napkins

shampoo and soaps

shaving cream

Nursing facilities are allowed to carry brand names of their choosing for these products.

Medications

acetaminophen

aspirin including buffered types

cough and cold preparations

epsom salts

glycerin suppositories

hydrogen peroxide

isopropyl alcohol

milk of magnesia

mineral oil or emulsions of mineral oil

multivitamins

povidone douches

povidone-iodine solutions

sterile lubricant

topical antiseptics

vinegar douches

vitamin A&D ointment, vitamin B_1, and vitamin B_6

white petroleum jelly

zinc oxide

Selection of brand names is up to the facility unless a generic or other brand is specified by the state.

OTHER SERVICES TYPICALLY COVERED BY MEDICAID

alcoholism treatment

chemical dependency treatment

chiropractic services

dental care

emergency ambulance services

family planning services

hearing services and hearing aids

hospital services

lab services not available at the facility

prescription drugs (the state may impose a "restricted formulary" limiting drugs or brands Medicaid will pay for)

mental health services

orthotics

physician services

podiatric services

prosthetics

radiology

vision services

A facility may make arrangements for these services. Other routine or daily services that residents in a long-term care facility require are also provided: laundry (but not dry cleaning), three meals and nutritious snacks each day, non-emergency transportation if requested by the physician for medical reasons and given prior authorization, and others. Most of the items listed above are covered in the daily rate paid to the nursing facility by Medicaid, known as the "per diem."

TYPICALLY COVERED FOOD AND RELATED SERVICES

dietary supplements, such as protein or fiber supplements

enteral feeding formulas (these may be subject to the restricted formulary) and supplies

nursing services associated with total parenteral nutrition (TPN) (this is when nutrients are administered by an IV route)

nutritious meals and snacks

special therapeutic diets

water solutions

Nursing facilities are not required to offer a restaurantlike variety of foods each day, but they must offer at least one alternative to the standard menu offering for each meal in order to accommodate individual tastes. Further, individual choices may be limited by dietary restrictions imposed for medical reasons; for example, calorie limitations imposed in diabetic diets or salt content limitations for cardiac conditions.

In some cases, Medicaid will pay what is known as a "bed hold" for the recipient in a nursing facility; that is, Medicaid may pay a fixed amount to the facility to hold a bed a set number of days for a recipient voluntarily leaving the facility for nonmedical reasons. Policies on this vary, subject to the rules of the state program. Generally, Medicaid will *not* pay to hold the bed if the resident is admitted to the hospital. The nursing facility will have policies related to bed hold and residents may pay to hold the bed on their own in circumstances where Medicaid will not cover the bed hold.

The facility is required to provide the consumer with a written listing of all services available in the facility and their charges. This includes a complete listing of services covered by Medicaid in that state and by Medicare. Some facilities may require the payment of a deposit at or prior to the time of admission. This is allowed if the individual seeking admission is paying privately for care. However, if the individual is covered by Medicaid or Medicare at the time of admission, the facility is *not* allowed to charge any deposit at the time of admission. If you become eligible for Medicaid coverage during your stay, the facility may be required to refund any deposit you paid at admission.

Note: Not all nursing facilities participate in the Medicaid program; thus some require private payment for services. The law does not compel a nursing facility to admit any individual; however, an individual who becomes Medicaid-eligible while at the facility, after a time in the hospital, may not be refused readmission. Knowing which facilities participate in Medicare and/or Medicaid in advance can greatly ease the process of placement in long-term care when the time comes, especially for consumers who know whether they qualify for Medicaid, Medicare, or both. That kind of preplacement planning is a great stress reducer. See chapter 5, "Choosing a Long-Term Care Facility," for more on this.

■

MEDICAID HOME AND COMMUNITY-BASED CARE

Since 1982, the Health Care Financing Administration (HCFA) has been granting specific waivers, known as "2176 waivers," permitting Medicaid coverage and reimbursement for home and community-based services provided to people who would otherwise need nursing home or other institutional care. This is an important alternative choice to individuals needing services but desiring to remain at home as long as possible. For people eligible for Medicaid benefits who live in localities covered by the waiver program, services such as adult day care, respite care, personal care, and case management services may be provided in an individual's home or other community-based setting. Services are available for individuals suffering from dementia (impairment of cognitive ability or the ability to think, reason, and problem solve), including dementia caused by Alzheimer's disease. Local home health or community services providers can supply more information and help you gain access to these services, or you can contact your state Medicaid office. See the directory to state Medicaid offices (appendix B) at the back of this guide.

Provisions of the Omnibus Reconciliation Act (OBRA) of 1990 allow states to provide home and community care to functionally disabled elderly, defined as financially eligible people age 65 or older who require substantial assistance performing two of three specified activities of daily living (ADLs) including toileting, transferring, and eating. The act establishes more liberal criteria for individuals with a primary or secondary diagnosis of Alzheimer's disease, who qualify if they require substantial assistance (including verbal reminding or physical cuing) or supervision in performing two of five specified activities of daily living (bathing, dressing, toileting, transferring, and eating). Unlike other Medicaid benefits, federal funds for this state option are capped at a specific level. Contact your state Medicaid office for availability of this program.

■

MEDICARE

The Medicare program is run and financed from the federal level and pays benefits to approximately 40 million Americans. Individuals age 65 and over and certain disabled individuals *under* the age of 65 are eligible for Medicare benefits. The parent agency responsible for processing claims, enforcing standards, and paying for services is the Health Care Financing Administration (HCFA), a division of the U.S. Department of Health and Human Services. Specific information, assistance, and applications for Medicare eligibility are available at your local Social Security Administration office. HCFA does not have local offices, operating regional offices only; however, they can direct you to the Social Security office nearest you by calling their toll-free information line at 1-(800) 772-1213.

Medicare is divided into three parts. **Part A** is hospital insurance, which helps pay for inpatient care in a hospital (acute care), inpatient care in a skilled nursing facility (SNF), kidney dialysis, home health care, and hospice care. **Part B,** medical insurance, helps pay for doctors' services, outpatient hospital services, durable medical equipment (walkers, commodes, oxygen equipment, etc.), and a number of other services and supplies not covered under Part A. **Part C,** known as **Medicare+Choice,** was created by the Balanced Budget Act of 1997 in sections 1851–1859 of the Social Security Act to provide more options, particularly for entry into managed care organizations, for Medicare beneficiaries. For more detail on Medicare Part C, see the "Balanced Budget Act Brings Changes to the Medicare Program" section later in this chapter.

Part A has deductibles and coinsurance (the amount of a covered service's cost that the consumer or insurer must pay), but most people do not have to pay monthly premiums. Part B has monthly premiums, coinsurance, and deductibles that must be paid by the consumer or through coverage by another insurance plan, such as Medigap (discussed later in this chapter). Premium, deductible, and coinsurance amounts are set each year based on formulas established by law. Recipients are notified of changes in these amounts annually. The coinsurance or "copay" amount is 20 percent of the Medicare-approved charges for most services.

The information that follows is drawn from HCFA publications *Medicare and You: Original Medicare Plan & Other Medicare Health Plan Choices* (1998) and the *Medicare Handbook* (1996, 1997). Access this information on the Internet at www.medicare.gov/publications/handbook.html or call 1-800-638-6833 (TTY,TDD: 1-800-820-1202).

ELIGIBILITY FOR MEDICARE PART A AND AUTOMATIC ENROLLMENT IN MEDICARE

In general, people age 65 and over are eligible for premium-free Medicare Part A benefits, based on their own or their spouse's employment. You qualify for premium-free Medicare Part A benefits if you are 65 years of age or older and *any* of the following three statements is true:

1. You receive benefits under the Social Security or Railroad Retirement system.

2. You could receive benefits under Social Security or the Railroad Retirement system but have not filed for them.

3. You or your spouse had Medicare-covered government employment.

Generally, if either you or your spouse worked for at least 10 years, you will be able to get premium-free Medicare Part A benefits. You can verify eligibility for Part A coverage by contacting your local Social Security Administration office to see if you or your spouse worked long enough under Social Security, Railroad Retirement, as a government employee, or a combination of these to qualify.

If you are already getting Social Security or Railroad Retirement benefits when you turn 65, you will automatically get a Medicare card in the mail. If you are disabled, you will automatically get a Medicare card in the mail when you have been a disability beneficiary under Social Security or Railroad Retirement for 24 months.

The Medicare card will show that you can get both Medicare Part A (hospital insurance that does not require a monthly premium payment) and Part B (medical insurance that *does* require the payment of a monthly premium). If you decide that you do not want Part B medical insurance, the card comes with instructions for declining that portion of Medicare coverage. Before deciding to decline that coverage, review the listing of covered supplies and services provided under Part B later in this chapter to be sure that you are comfortable going without that coverage.

If you are *under age 65* and you have been a disabled beneficiary under Social Security or the Railroad Retirement Board for more than 24 months, you qualify for premium-free Part A benefits. You must apply at the Social Security office as soon as you become disabled.

Finally, individuals under age 65 may qualify for premium-free Part A benefits if they require kidney dialysis for permanent kidney failure or if they have had a kidney transplant. To order a copy of *Medicare Coverage of Kidney Dialysis and Kidney Transplant Services* write the Consumer Information Center, Department 33, Pueblo, CO 81009, and request publication 594B.

HOW TO APPLY FOR MEDICARE WHEN ENROLLMENT IS NOT AUTOMATIC

Individuals in the special eligibility circumstances just described and individuals who have not applied for Social Security or Railroad Retirement benefits or individuals in certain government employment may *not* automatically be enrolled in Medicare and get a card in the mail. These individuals must file an application for Medicare benefits. The first step is to check with the Social Security Administration office to see if you can get Medicare under the Social Security system or based on Medicare-covered government employment. Check with the Railroad Retirement office if you are able to get Medicare under the Railroad Retirement system.

If you must apply for Medicare, the application should be made during the "initial enrollment period" to avoid late enrollment surcharges that may apply. See the section called "Buying Medicare Part A and B" later in this chapter for more details on late enrollment. The initial enrollment period is a seven-month period that starts three months *before* the month you first qualify for Medicare. **Warning:** If you do not sign up for Medicare during the first three months of your initial enrollment period, there will be a delay of from one to three months in the start of your Part B coverage. If you do not enroll at any time during your initial enrollment period, you will not be able to enroll at all until the next general enrollment period unless you qualify for a special enrollment period. A general enrollment period is held each year from January 1 to March 31, and when

enrollment takes place during this period, coverage does not begin until July 1 of the year of enrollment.

ELIGIBILITY FOR MEDICARE PART B

Most U.S. citizens 65 years of age and over are eligible for Medicare Part B benefits; in general, anyone who qualifies for premium-free Medicare Part A benefits based on work can enroll for Part B benefits. In any case, the monthly premiums must be paid in order to receive Part B benefits.

BUYING MEDICARE PART A AND PART B

An individual who does not have enough work credits or whose spouse does not have enough work credits to be able to get Medicare Part A benefits and who is over the age of 65 may be able to buy Medicare Part A and Part B or Part B only by paying the monthly premiums. Also, it is possible to buy Medicare Parts A and B if you are disabled and lost your premium-free Part A coverage because you are working.

Some individuals 65 or older have Medicare Medical Insurance (Part B) but do not have the 40 quarters of work credits of Social Security coverage to qualify for premium-free Part A. For individuals in this situation, Part A is available by paying a monthly premium. This is referred to as "premium hospital insurance."

If you or your spouse has fewer than 30 quarters of Social Security work credits, your Part A premium will be over $261 a month. If you have more than 30 quarters but less than 40 quarters of work credit, the monthly premium will be more than $183. The premium amounts are adjusted annually and your area Social Security office can give you the prevailing rate at the time you apply.

The general enrollment period for Part A runs from January 1 to March 31 each year. It is important to enroll in the Medicare program as soon as you become eligible, since the monthly premium may be 10 percent *higher* if you enroll more than one year *after* you became eligible (reached age 65) to buy Part A. Also, it is important to remember that your coverage does not begin until July 1 of the year you enroll.

If you have premium-free hospital insurance (Part A) but do not have Part B medical insurance, you can sign up for Part B during a general enrollment period. As with Part A enrollment, the Part B general enrollment period runs from January 1 to March 31 each year. Your coverage will begin on July 1 of the year in which you enroll. As with the Part A general enrollment period, a 10 percent premium surcharge may be applied to your premiums for each 12-month period you could have had Part B but were not enrolled.

Individuals who have been covered by a group health insurance plan based on their own or their spouse's current employment sometimes do not enroll in Medicare. Delayed enrollment in Medicare Parts A and B without a surcharge or waiting for the general enrollment period is generally available if you are covered by a group health plan (not a retirement medical plan) at the time you are first eligible for Medicare. This situation is covered by a "special enrollment period."

For individuals age 65 or over, the special enrollment period to enroll in Part B lasts seven months starting with the month

1. Your (or your spouse's) employment ends, or

2. Your coverage under the employer group health plan ends,

whichever comes first.

The seven-month special enrollment period also applies under certain circumstances if you are disabled and covered by a group health plan based on your current employment or a family member's current employment. In that situation, you may enroll in Medicare Part B during the seven-month period that begins

1. When the current employment ends,

2. When the group health plan is no longer classifiable as a large group health plan, which under federal rules is one that covers 100 or more employees, or

3. When the group health plan coverage is terminated.

Be sure to contact your local Social Security Administration office as soon as employment ends or your group health insurance coverage ends to obtain Part B enrollment materials.

THE MEDICARE CARD

The Medicare card shows your name as you will be identified by the Medicare system, your individual health insurance claim number, the date your coverage began, and which parts of Medicare you have. It is important to use your name as it appears on the card on all claims and correspondence sent to Medicare; that is, if the card shows a middle initial, that is how it should appear on any claims or correspondence. If there is any error in your name as it appears on your card, notify the Social Security office as soon as possible to get it corrected and have a new card issued.

The health insurance claim number that appears on the card is used for claiming benefits under both parts of Medicare. It usually is a nine-digit number followed by one or two letters. There may also be another number after the letter. As with your name, the full claim number must always be used as it appears on the card on any claims or correspondence sent to Medicare. When a husband and wife both have Medicare, they will receive separate cards and have their own claim numbers. When you receive your Medicare card, it may be useful to make a few photocopies of it to keep for reference or emergency use in the event your original card becomes lost, but if you do lose your original card, you should still contact the Social Security office to have a new card sent to you.

Always carry your Medicare card with you and present it when you receive health care services, but do not use it until *after* the effective date which appears on it. *Do not let anyone else use your Medicare card.*

MEDICARE DOES NOT COVER EVERYTHING

Medicare covers a wide array of supplies and services for the medical and nursing care of many health conditions, but by law it is restricted from paying for certain services. These include the following:

1. Care services provided by immediate relatives or members of your own household. However, if you happen to have a relative who is a licensed health care professional (e.g., RN, LPN, or certified nurse's aide) who works for a licensed home health or hospice agency that is a provider that participates in the Medicare program, that relative may provide care to you. In such a case, only the agency can bill Medicare and get paid for the care the relative provides.

2. Services covered under other government programs for which you may be eligible.

3. Custodial care—assistance with bathing, walking, bed mobility, repositioning, dressing, eating, and medication administration—when that is the only type of care you require. Care is considered custodial in nature when it may be provided safely and reasonably by people without professional skills or training.

4. Care that is not reasonable and medically necessary under Medicare program standards to treat an illness or injury. This means Medicare will not pay for any experimental or investigational treatment of an illness, any treatment not approved by the Food and Drug Administration (FDA), any treatment not appropriate for your diagnosis or condition, or care or treatment rendered more often than is necessary to treat your condition or in a setting that is inappropriate for the treatment of your condition. For example, if the physician writes an order to admit you to a skilled nursing facility when the type of care you require could be rendered at home or by an outpatient care facility, Medicare may render a decision *not* to pay for the care. Or, for example, if you stay in a skilled nursing facility beyond the point in your care when skilled nursing is medically necessary, Medicare payments will end at the point when skilled nursing was no longer required. Each claim is reviewed by Medicare intermediaries on a case-by-case basis.

5. Care provided outside the United States. It is important to note that Puerto Rico, Guam, American Samoa, the Northern Mariana Islands, and the U.S. Virgin Islands are considered part of the United States. If you are planning to travel outside the United States, it may be advisable to buy short-term health insurance that would cover you during your foreign travel. In some rare instances, Medicare may cover care provided in Canada or Mexico. Generally, this will happen only when a Canadian or Mexican hospital that can provide care for your condition is closer than a U.S. hospital, particularly in an emergency situation. Generally, Medicare will also pay for physician and ambulance services provided in Canada or Mexico in connection with a covered inpatient hospital stay.

When Medicare does not cover a service or item, it issues a statement called a "denial," which notes that it will not cover the service or item and explains why.

WHAT HAPPENS WHEN MEDICARE DOES NOT PAY

In some cases, when Medicare denies payment for your claim, you will not be held responsible for paying the provider. This can occur under a portion of the Medicare law known as the "limitation on liability." This proviso applies only when *all three* of the following conditions are met:

1. The services are provided by an institutional provider, such as a hospital, skilled nursing facility, or home health agency that participates in Medicare, or a doctor or other supplier who accepts assignment (accepts the price limits set by Medicare for their services as payment in full for those services).

2. Medicare denied your claim for *one* of the following reasons:

   ■ The care was custodial in nature.

   ■ The care was not reasonable or medically necessary.

   ■ For home health services, the patient was not truly "homebound" or did not require skilled nursing on an intermittent basis.

- The only reason for the denial is that, in error, you were placed in a skilled nursing facility bed that was not approved by Medicare.

3. You did not know or you could not reasonably be expected to know that Medicare does not cover the services you were given. For example, you did not know because you were not given written notice at the time of admission to the facility, as is required by law.

The limitation on liability provision does *not* apply to Medicare Part B services provided by a doctor or supplier who did not accept assignment of the claim. However, in certain situations Medicare law protects you from paying for doctor services provided on a nonassigned basis that are denied as "not reasonable and necessary." If your doctor knows or should know that a treatment is likely to be denied by Medicare as not reasonable or necessary, he or she must, before performing the treatment or service, give you written notice that Medicare will probably not pay for the service and why. You must also agree in writing to pay for the service before you can be held responsible to pay for it in the event of a denial by Medicare.

If you did not receive this notice, you are *not* required to pay for the service. If you did pay for the service but did not receive such a notice, you may be entitled to a refund from the doctor. It's important to remember that the doctor's written notice is not the same as an official determination by Medicare. If you disagree with it, ask your doctor to submit a claim to Medicare for an official determination.

If you receive a bill from a doctor, supplier, or other health care provider for a service denied by Medicare and you believe the limitation on liability applies, contact your Medicare carrier on how to handle the bill.

WHAT MEDICARE PART A HOSPITAL INSURANCE DOES COVER

Medicare Part A pays for four types of medically necessary care:

1. Inpatient hospital care.

2. Inpatient care in a skilled nursing facility following a hospital stay of at least three days duration.

3. Home health care.

4. Hospice care.

Medicare Part A helps pay for inpatient hospital care when *all* the following conditions are met:

1. A doctor orders the inpatient hospital care.

2. The care you require can be provided *only* in a hospital.

3. The hospital is participating in Medicare or the care is required on an emergency basis but is provided in a nonparticipating facility.

4. The utilization review committee of the hospital, a peer review organization (PRO), or an intermediary does not disapprove your stay.

MAJOR SERVICES COVERED UNDER PART A

During inpatient hospital care, Medicare Part A covers the following:

1. A semiprivate room (two to four beds in a room).

2. All meals including special diets.

3. Regular nursing services.

4. Costs associated with special care units such as intensive care or coronary care.

5. Drugs furnished by the hospital during your stay.

6. Whole blood, packed red blood cells, blood components, and the cost of blood processing and administration of blood transfusions.

7. Lab tests included in your hospital bill.

8. X-rays and other radiology services, including radiation therapy billed by the hospital.

9. Medical supplies such as casts, surgical dressings, and splints.

10. Use of appliances or assistive devices (walkers or wheelchairs, for example).

11. Operating and recovery room costs.

12. Rehabilitation services, such as physical therapy, occupational therapy, and speech therapy.

13. Care in a psychiatric hospital. A special lifetime limit of a total of 190 days of care applies to Part A coverage for this type of care. However, psychiatric care rendered in a general hospital is *not* subject to the 190-day limitation and is treated the same as other Medicare inpatient hospital care.

14. Care in a Christian Science sanitorium if it is operated or listed and certified by the First Church of Christ, Scientist, in Boston, but Medicare Part B will not pay for the practitioner.

Some items that are *not* covered by Medicare Part A as a part of inpatient hospital care include:

1. Personal convenience items you may request such as a telephone or television in the room.

2. Private duty nursing.

3. Any extra charges for a private room unless a private room is medically necessary, for isolation, for example.

Note: Physician services are not covered under Part A. Physician services are covered under Part B.

*BENEFIT PERIOD, DEDUCTIBLE, AND COINSURANCE
FOR ACUTE CARE UNDER PART A*

"Benefit periods" are the way Medicare measures your use of services under Medicare Part A. Your first benefit period begins the first time you receive inpatient hospital care after your hospital insurance coverage begins. If the care required meets the four qualifying conditions listed earlier in this section, Part A will pay for up to 90 days of medically necessary inpatient hospital care per benefit period. Remember that a deductible does apply to the hospital insurance portion of Medicare. In 1997, for example, the deductible was $760. The deductible must be paid only once per benefit period. A coinsurance amount must be paid by the consumer after the 60th day of acute care. In 1997, that amount was $190 per day. A benefit period begins when you are admitted to the hospital for inpatient care and ends when you have not received inpatient care, skilled nursing, or covered rehabilitation services for 60 consecutive days. There is no limit to the number of benefit periods you can have for hospital or skilled nursing care.

If you must be in the hospital more than 90 consecutive days, Medicare provides for what are known as **reserve days.** Each recipient is allowed a maximum of 60 reserve days in his or her lifetime. Each time a reserve day is used, it is deducted from the total of 60 days available to the individual and only the remaining total is available for use. For example, if an individual uses five reserve days during a hospital stay (hospitalization for a total of 95 consecutive days), then only 55 reserve days remain available even if a new benefit period starts. A coinsurance amount applies in the reserve-day period. Remember, these deductibles and copays are adjusted (generally upward, of course) annually. You decide when to use your reserve days. If you *do not* wish to use your reserve days, however, you must notify the hospital in writing. This can be done anytime from the date of admission to up to 90 days after discharge from the hospital.

SKILLED NURSING CARE

Medicare Parts A and B will help pay for care in a skilled nursing facility if *all seven* of the following conditions are met:

1. The facility must be a participant in the Medicare program.

2. Your condition must require daily skilled nursing or

skilled rehabilitation services that, as a practical matter, can be provided only in a skilled nursing facility.

3. You must have been in the hospital at least three days in a row, not including the day of discharge, prior to your admission to the skilled nursing facility.

4. Admission to the skilled nursing facility occurred within 30 days of your discharge from the hospital.

5. Your care in the skilled nursing facility is for a condition that was treated in the hospital, or for a condition that arose while you were receiving care in the skilled nursing facility for a condition that was treated in the hospital.

6. A medical professional certifies that you require and receive skilled nursing or rehabilitation services on a daily basis.

7. The Medicare intermediary does not disapprove your stay.

It is important to remember that Medicare Part A will *not* help pay for skilled care that is required less than daily or for care that is considered custodial in nature when that is the only type of care required. Again, custodial care is the type of care that does not require the skills of a professional nurse or therapist for performance or observation: bathing, dressing, walking, toileting, bed mobility, eating, grooming, taking medicine, and the like. Of course, when skilled nursing or rehabilitation *is* required, the custodial type of care is covered as a part of the skilled facility stay.

When you are in a nursing home, Medicare Part A will help pay for the following services:

1. A semiprivate room (two to four beds in a room).

2. All your meals, including special diets and nutritious snacks provided by the facility.

3. Regular nursing services.

4. Physical, speech, and occupational therapy.

5. Drugs furnished by the facility.

6. Blood, blood products, and transfusion costs.

7. Medical supplies such as casts, splints, restraints, postural devices, pressure relief cushions, positioning pillows, and other equipment that is furnished by the facility.

8. Use of appliances and assistive devices such as canes, walkers, and wheelchairs furnished by the facility. It must be understood that most of these items are and remain the property of the facility—but since the law requires the facility make these things available to residents who need them, the *facility* can get reimbursed for acquiring them.

As with Medicare coverage for acute care, some of the same things are *not* covered as a part of Medicare coverage for care in a skilled nursing facility. Some of the things not covered as part of skilled nursing care include:

1. Personal convenience items you might request such as a television or telephone.

2. Private duty nurses.

3. Any extra charges for a private room, unless it is determined to be medically necessary.

Physician services are not covered under Part A. Those services are covered under Part B.

BENEFIT PERIOD AND COINSURANCE AMOUNTS FOR SKILLED NURSING

Benefit periods for long-term care in a skilled nursing facility are similar to benefit periods for acute (hospital) care with some important differences. The benefit period begins when the individual is admitted for care to the skilled nursing facility. Medicare will help pay for up to 100 days of skilled nursing facility care per benefit period. In each benefit period, Part A pays for *all* covered services (no coinsurance must be paid by the consumer) for the first 20 days of care. However, for the 21st day to the 100th day, there is a coinsurance amount that will have to be paid by the consumer. There is no deductible for skilled nursing care.

If you leave a skilled nursing facility and are readmitted within 30 days, it is not necessary to have another three-day hospital stay for your skilled nursing care to be covered. If you have days remaining from the total 100 days available per benefit period and you require skilled care for the condition that you were originally treated for in the skilled facility, Medicare will help pay for your care.

Note: The skilled nursing facility may *not* charge you a deposit as a condition of admission when your care will be covered by Medicare. If, during your stay in the skilled nursing facility, the facility's staff determines you no longer require skilled nursing[1] or rehabilitative care, they must notify you of that change in your status immediately. You can request that the facility submit this decision to Medicare for review and a final determination if you disagree with the facility's decision. The facility may not charge you a deposit until Medicare issues its determination in the matter. You will have to pay any coinsurance amounts due and for any noncovered services while your claim is being processed.

HOME HEALTH SERVICES

A long-term care option that is rapidly growing in popularity is home health care. Home health agencies deliver skilled nursing, aide, and therapy services in the patient's own home. Medicare will help pay for those services if all four of the following conditions are met:

1. You require intermittent skilled nursing or therapy such as speech, occupational, or physical therapy.

2. You are confined to your own home (homebound). This means that you are not independently mobile in the community, such as being able to drive to other loca-

tions for care. Generally, some limited activity outdoors in the immediate vicinity of one's residence does not alter the finding that one is homebound.

3. You are under the care of a physician, there is a doctor's order for home health care, and the physician sets up or approves a home health care plan for you.

4. The home health agency providing care participates in Medicare.

Home health services are covered under Medicare Part A *and* under Part B for individuals who do not have Part A. If all four of the above conditions are met, Medicare will pay for the following home health services through provisions of either Part A or Part B:

1. Part-time or intermittent skilled nursing care. This can include up to eight hours per day of medically necessary nursing care for up to 21 consecutive days or, in certain circumstances, even longer.

2. Physical therapy, speech therapy, occupational therapy, or a combination of these if medically necessary. When you no longer require skilled nursing, physical therapy, or speech therapy, Medicare will continue to pay for home health services if you continue to need occupational therapy.

3. Part-time or intermittent nurse aide services if skilled nursing or skilled therapy services are being provided.

4. Medical social services. (See chapter 14 for a general description.)

5. Medical supplies.

6. Durable medical equipment such as a walker, cane, wheelchair, or hospital bed. (Medicare will pay 80 percent of the approved amount.)

---

1. **Skilled level of care** means the person required daily observations by a nurse because of unstable conditions or possibility of complications; skilled care management because of complex or multiple conditions; or daily skilled services such as restorative nursing, patient teaching, physical therapy, or speech therapy; or complex nursing care such as wound care or IV therapy.

Home health services that are not covered by Medicare include:

1. Twenty-four-hour-a-day nursing care in the patient's home.

2. Drugs and biologicals.

3. Meals delivered to the patient's home.

4. Homemaker services, laundry services, meal preparation, shopping services, chore services, nonemergency transportation, or personal care worker services.

5. Blood transfusions. (These are covered under Part B when done on an outpatient basis at a hospital and are billed by the hospital.)

To determine if you would qualify for home health services under Medicare, ask your physician or the social worker at the facility you are being discharged from to refer you to a Medicare participating home health agency. The agency will review your case to determine if Medicare requirements for coverage are met. The home health agency should not charge for this evaluation.

BENEFIT PERIOD AND DEDUCTIBLE AND COINSURANCE AMOUNTS FOR HOME HEALTH CARE

There is no specific benefit period for coverage of home health services. That is, as long as the qualifying conditions are being met, coverage will continue. Medicare pays 100 percent of covered costs with no coinsurance amount passed on to the consumer. As mentioned earlier, Medicare pays 80 percent of the approved cost for durable medical equipment. There is no deductible for home health care services. You may be charged only for services or supplies not covered by Medicare.

The Balanced Budget Act signed into law in August 1997 reduced Medicare spending on home health benefits by an estimated $16.2 billion over the subsequent five years. The impact on home health was so significant that in October 1998 the appropriations budget for 1999 restored over a billion dollars in funding. Despite the added funding, the effects of a prospective payment system for Medicare home health services will be felt as the new century begins.

HOSPICE CARE

Although traditionally a hospice has been thought of as a facility that serves individuals who are terminally ill, hospice care can be provided in the home as well as in an inpatient setting. Hospice care is generally directed toward relieving pain, treating symptoms of the terminal condition, offering comfort measures and supportive care for the patient and his or her family. It may include certain services that generally are not otherwise provided under Medicare.

Medicare Part A will help pay for hospice care if *all three* of the following conditions are met:

1. A doctor certifies that the patient is terminally ill.

2. The patient chooses to receive care from a hospice instead of the standard Medicare benefits for the terminal illness.

3. Care is provided by a hospice agency that participates in the Medicare program.

Medicare will help pay for the following hospice services when provided by or through a Medicare-participating hospice agency:

1. Nursing services up to daily, if needed.

2. Physician services.

3. Home health aide, custodial care, and homemaker services on a daily basis, if needed.

4. Drugs, including outpatient treatments for pain relief and symptom management.

5. Physical therapy, occupational therapy, and speech/language pathology.

6. Medical social services.

7. Medical supplies and appliances.

8. Short-term inpatient care, including respite care. Respite care is provided in a facility other than the patient's own home, allowing the person who regularly assists with the patient's home care—generally the spouse or other family member such as a son or daughter—time to rest. Each inpatient respite care stay is limited to a total of five days in a row.

If a patient requires treatment for a condition not related to the terminal illness while receiving hospice care, Medicare will continue to pay for all necessary covered services under the standard Medicare benefit program.

Note: The Medicare Part A hospice benefit will *not* pay for treatments other than those for pain relief and symptom management of a terminal illness. However, other portions of Medicare will generally help pay for treatments not related to the terminal illness. More detailed information is available in the free booklet *Medicare: Hospice Benefits.* (Request publication 591B from the Consumer Information Center, Department 33, Pueblo CO 81009.)

The Balanced Budget Act of 1997 changed services covered in the hospice benefit, effective April 1, 1998. It provided that Medicare services in addition to those specifically required are covered hospice services when they are included in the plan of care.

BENEFIT PERIOD AND DEDUCTIBLE AND COINSURANCE AMOUNTS FOR HOSPICE CARE

Special benefit periods applying to hospice care differ from those for acute and long-term care. Part A covers care for two 90-day periods, followed by an unlimited number of 60-day periods.

If the beneficiary cancels hospice care during any of the first three benefit periods, any days left in that period are lost. The days left in any remaining benefit periods are still available. Also, it is possible to disenroll from hospice care during any benefit period, return to regular Medicare coverage, and later reenter hospice care if another benefit period is available. If you elect to cancel hospice care during the final extension period, the Medicare hospice benefit will *not* be available to you again.

No deductible applies to the hospice care benefit. Medicare pays for all covered services under the hospice benefit. A 5 percent coinsurance amount applies to the cost of outpatient drugs, up to a maximum of $5 for each prescription. The 5 percent coinsurance amount applies to the cost of inpatient respite care as well.

PROVIDERS AND PAYMENT UNDER PART A

Providers—hospitals, skilled nursing facilities, home health agencies, and hospices—bill you for any part of the deductible you have not met and any coinsurance payment you may owe.

When the provider sends Medicare a Part A claim for payment, you will get a "notice of utilization" that explains the decision Medicare has made on the claim. Remember that this is not a bill. Any questions you have on the content of the notice should be directed to the address on the face of the notice. Payment for the billed services will be made by Medicare directly to the provider for you.

WHAT MEDICARE PART B MEDICAL INSURANCE DOES COVER

Medicare Part B medical insurance coverage helps pay for the following:

1. Doctors' services.

2. Outpatient hospital care.

3. Diagnostic tests.

4. Durable medical equipment.

5. Emergency ambulance services.

6. Numerous other services and supplies not covered by Medicare Part A.

It may be beneficial to consider some of these broad areas of coverage in more detail.

Part B medical insurance will help pay for physicians' and certain other specialists' care provided in an office, a hospital, a skilled nursing facility, your home, or virtually any other location. Specific services covered include:

1. Medical and surgical services, including anesthesia.

2. Diagnostic tests and procedures that are part of your treatment.

3. Radiology and pathology services provided by doctors while you are an inpatient in the hospital or on an outpatient basis.

4. Treatment of mental illness, including treatment by nonphysicians such as psychologists and social workers. The care can be provided in various settings including hospitals, skilled nursing facilities, community mental health centers, and comprehensive outpatient rehabilitation facilities. When furnished on an outpatient basis, mental health services are subject to a payment limitation. Once the annual deductible ($100.00) is met, Medicare Part B pays 50 percent of the approved amount for these services. On assigned claims (where the provider accepts assignment, which is the allowable Medicare rate), the beneficiary is responsible for paying the remaining 50 percent. On unassigned claims, the beneficiary may have to pay more. (See the section on assignment later in this chapter.) Partial hospitalization for treatment of mental illness or brief office visits for the purpose of monitoring or changing medications are not subject to this payment limitation.

5. X-rays.

6. Services of your doctor's office nurse.

7. Drugs and biologicals that cannot be self-administered.

8. Transfusions of whole blood and blood components.

9. Medical supplies.

10. Physical/occupational therapy and speech pathology services.

11. A second opinion by another physician when your doctor recommends surgery and a third physician's opinion when the first two opinions contradict each other.

12. Chiropractor's services to treat subluxation (dislocation) of a vertebra of the spine by manual manipulation. This is the only chiropractic service covered by Part B.

13. Annual mammograms.

14. Pap tests and pelvic exams every three years or annually if abnormalities appeared in past three years.

15. Annual prostate cancer screening.

16. Colorectal cancer screening: fecal occult blood tests annually, flexible sigmoidoscopy every four years, colonoscopy every two years (if high risk), or barium enema in place of colonoscopy or sigmoidoscopy.

17. Diabetes self-management.

18. Bone density measurement (frequency depends on your health status).

19. Some immunizations, such as flu and pneumonia shots and hepatitis B immunization for individuals considered at high or intermediate risk for contracting the disease. If the entity providing the vaccine and administering it accept assignment, there will be no cost to you; if they do not, there may be a charge to you in addition to the Medicare-approved amount. Flu shots are annual. Pneumonia vaccines are generally given once. Hepatitis B vaccine is given in a series of three shots. Booster doses are generally not needed.

Physician's services *not* covered by Medicare Part B include:

1. Most routine physical examinations and tests directly related to such examinations.

2. Most routine foot care and dental care. Medicare Part B will help pay for podiatrists' services to treat injuries and diseases of the foot, such as ingrown toenails, hammer toe deformities, bunion deformities, and heel

spurs. Routine foot care, such as cutting nails, removal of corns or calluses, and hygienic care, is generally *not* covered unless you are under a doctor's care for a condition affecting your legs or feet such as peripheral vascular disease or diabetes. Part B does *not* pay for care in connection with filling, removal of, or replacement of teeth; root canal therapy; surgery for impacted teeth; or other surgical procedures involving the teeth or structures supporting the teeth. However, Medicare will help pay for care by a dentist when the medical problem is more extensive than the teeth or their supporting structures. Part A will help pay for the inpatient care if the care requires hospitalization even if the dental care itself is not covered by Medicare.

3. Examinations for fitting or prescribing eyeglasses or hearing aids. However, Medicare will help pay for cataract spectacles, cataract contact lenses, or intra-ocular lenses (implant) that replace the natural lens in cataract surgery. Medicare will also pay for one pair of conventional eyeglasses or contact lenses if necessary after cataract surgery with the insertion of an intraocular lens.

4. Some immunizations.

5. Most prescription drugs; however, Medicare does help pay for the following:

   ■ Antigens, under certain circumstances.

   ■ Blood and blood products.

   ■ E-poietin alpha for dialysis patients (stimulates red blood cell production).

   ■ Hemophilia clotting factors and items necessary for self-administration.

   ■ Immunosuppressive drugs (given to prevent transplanted organ rejection) for at least one year from the date of discharge after organ transplantation.

   ■ Certain oral antineoplastic (anticancer) drugs.

6. Cosmetic surgery unless it is necessary as a result of accidental injury or to improve the function of a malformed part of the body.

Medicare Part B will help pay for services provided by the following nonphysician practitioners if they are approved by Medicare for services for which they accept assignment:

1. Certified registered nurse anesthetist (CRNA).

2. Certified nurse midwife.

3. Clinical psychologist.

4. Clinical social worker.

5. Physician assistant.

6. Nurse practitioner and clinical nurse specialist in collaboration with a physician.

Some of these practitioners are approved to render their services only in certain facilities, and it is advisable to ask your Medicare carrier if Medicare will help pay for their services in your particular situation.

OUTPATIENT HOSPITAL SERVICES COVERED BY MEDICARE PART B

The following listing covers some of the major outpatient hospital care Part B will help pay for. You must meet the $100 deductible before Part B kicks in and you must also pay a 20 percent coinsurance amount for covered care. Covered services include:

1. Services in an emergency room or outpatient clinic, including same day surgery.

2. Laboratory tests billed by the hospital.

3. Portable diagnostic X-rays.

4. Pap smear screening for cervical cancer.

6. Radiation therapy.

7. Kidney dialysis and transplantation.

8. Heart and liver transplants in certain situations. Contact your HMO or Medicare carrier regarding coverage if such transplants may be necessary.

9. Local emergency ambulance transportation to a hospital or skilled nursing facility, if the ambulance, equipment, and staff meet Medicare requirements, and transportation in any other vehicle could endanger your health. Air ambulance service can be covered only if significant risk of death or serious health impact exists if treatment is delayed and land ambulance service is not available or would be too time-consuming. If an air ambulance was used inappropriately (use of a land ambulance would not have jeopardized your health), Medicare will pay for the ambulance, but *at the land ambulance rate.* You are then responsible for the difference in cost.

Some outpatient hospital services *not* covered by Medicare Part B include:

1. Most routine physical examinations and tests directly related to such exams.

2. Eye or ear exams to prescribe or fit glasses or hearing aids.

3. Most prescription drugs.

4. Most routine foot care.

DURABLE MEDICAL EQUIPMENT COVERED UNDER MEDICARE PART B

Durable medical equipment (DME) includes walkers, canes, wheelchairs, hospital beds, oxygen equipment, suction machines, IV pumps, enteral feeding pumps, and so on. Medicare will pay 80 percent of the approved amount for durable medical equipment if the following conditions are met:

1. It must be ordered by a physician for use in your own home and it must be medically necessary. Nursing or

rehabilitation centers are not considered your own home.

2. The equipment must be reusable.

3. The equipment must serve primarily a medical purpose.

4. It must not be of use to people who are not ill or injured.

5. It must be appropriate for use in your home.

Be aware that some equipment must be rented—IV and enteral feeding pumps, for example—while other equipment is purchased; some items may be rented or purchased. Durable medical equipment suppliers fall under rules enacted as of October 1, 1993, which are designed to prevent misuse or fraud in the DME market. Some of the key requirements include:

1. Suppliers must be approved by Medicare and have a Medicare supplier number. If you purchase or rent equipment from a DME supplier who is not approved, Medicare may not pay your claim.

2. Suppliers may not *initiate* communication with you by phone or mail to offer to get your doctor to approve an item. They may, however, contact you in response to a request made by your doctor or other health care provider such as a home health agency.

3. Suppliers cannot say they work for or represent Medicare.

4. Suppliers may not deliver any equipment to your home that was not ordered by your doctor or by you.

5. They may not supply used equipment to you and then bill it as a new item to Medicare.

6. The supplier cannot offer to provide equipment to you at no cost or offer to pay your coinsurance amount for you. This practice is illegal.

If a DME supplier engages in any of these practices, notify your Medicare carrier. You do not submit claims to Medicare for durable medical equipment—suppliers do that. They submit their bill to one of four regional carriers that handle all DME, supplies, prosthetics, and orthotics claims for Medicare. See appendix E at the back of this guide for the addresses of these regional carriers.

ORTHOTIC, PROSTHETIC, AND ORTHOPEDIC ITEMS COVERED UNDER PART B

An **orthotic device** is one that acts as a brace or support for a body part to prevent deformity, maintain proper body alignment, or preserve function. Wrist splints, neck supports, and postural devices are examples. A **prosthesis** is an artificial body part used to achieve function or appearance. Examples of prosthetic devices are artificial limbs, eyes, and breasts. Included in this coverage are ostomy bags and supplies; breast prostheses and surgical brassiere after mastectomy; eye, arm, or leg prostheses; and arm, leg, or back braces. Orthopedic shoes are not covered unless they are an integral part of a leg brace and the cost is included in the charge for the braces. Denture plates and partial dentures are not covered.

Therapeutic shoes or inserts for individuals with severe diabetic foot disease *are* covered (one pair per calendar year) in this benefit if ordered by a physician and provided and fitted by a podiatrist, orthotist, or prosthetist.

OTHER SERVICES AND SUPPLIES COVERED BY MEDICARE

1. **Ambulatory Surgical Services.** Medicare will help pay for certain approved surgical procedures performed at an ambulatory surgical center that participates in the Medicare program. Ambulatory surgery is a minor surgical procedure that is often done under local anesthesia; generally the patient goes home the day the procedure is performed. In addition to helping to pay for the procedure, Medicare will also help pay for the physician's services and anesthesia in connection with the procedure.

2. **Comprehensive Outpatient Rehabilitation Facility Services.** Medicare will help pay for services provided by a Medicare-participating comprehensive outpatient rehabilitation facility (CORF) under certain circumstances. For coverage to be obtained, you must be referred to the CORF by a physician who certifies that you need skilled rehabilitation services. Services that are covered include the following:

a. Physicians' services.

b. Physical therapy.

c. Speech therapy.

d. Occupation therapy.

e. Respiratory therapy.

f. Counseling.

g. Related services.

There is a 20 percent coinsurance amount for CORF services and the annual deductible ($100) would also apply. Mental health services provided in a CORF setting would have the same limitations on coverage listed on page 29.

3. **Rural Health Clinic Services.** Medicare will help pay for the following services provided by participating rural health clinics, subject to the 20 percent coinsurance and annual deductible:

a. Physicians' services.

b. Nurse practitioners' services.

c. Physician assistants' services.

d. Nurse midwives.

e. Clinical psychologists.

f. Clinical social workers.

g. Visiting nurse services under certain circumstances.

4. Federally Qualified Health Center Services. The services that may be obtained and covered by Medicare at a federally qualified health center are essentially the same as those at a rural health clinic as listed above. However, there are some important differences between the two. The federally qualified health center can provide certain *preventive* services (the center you have access to can tell you what services are part of the federal health center benefit), and you do *not* have to meet the annual Part B deductible ($100) at these centers although you would usually have to pay the 20 percent coinsurance amount. There are some exceptions to this as well; in certain cases, part or all of the coinsurance amount may be waived under Public Health Service guidelines.

5. Drugs and Biologicals. Although Medicare will *not* pay for most outpatient prescription drugs, Medicare will help pay for the following:

a. Antigens prepared by your physician (under certain circumstances). Ask your Medicare carrier if your antigens will be covered. Regional carriers are listed in appendix D at the back of the book.

b. Blood and blood components. Medicare will *not* pay for the first three unreplaced pints of blood.

c. E-poietin alpha for dialysis patients when it is self-administered or administered by a caregiver.

d. Hemophilia clotting factors and items related to their administration when the patient can use them without medical supervision to control bleeding.

e. Hepatitis B vaccine for individuals considered to be at high or intermediate risk for contracting hepatitis.

f. Immunosuppressive drugs used to prevent organ rejection following transplantation. Part B will pay for such therapy for more than a year.

g. Influenza and pneumococcal pneumonia vaccines.

h. Certain oral antineoplastic (anticancer) drugs.

At the heart of the Medicare Part B payment system is a fee schedule that lists the amount that Medicare will approve as charges for various services by providers. Medicare pays 80 percent of the approved amount found on the fee schedule for each service. Medicare will pay 80 percent of the doctor's fee for a service instead of the amount found on the fee schedule if the doctor's rate is lower than that found on the fee schedule. In general, the Medicare fee schedule is the lower of the two.

When a physician agrees to accept the amount approved by the Medicare carrier as the total payment for covered services, it is said that the physician "takes assignment." The assignment method is intended to save the consumer some money. When the physician or supplier submits a claim to Medicare, Medicare will pay 80 percent of the approved amount for the service or item supplied after subtracting the $100 deductible, if it has not already been met. The provider can charge you *only* for the remaining 20 percent of the approved amount and any portion of the deductible that Medicare did not pay. The provider can also charge you for any goods or services provided which are *not* covered by Medicare.

Providers and suppliers *must accept assignment* on all claims for services provided to Medicare beneficiaries who are eligible for Medicaid (medical assistance) through their state Medicaid program, including qualified medicare beneficiaries.

QUALIFIED MEDICARE BENEFICIARIES

In some cases, state Medicaid programs pay Medicare costs for elderly and disabled people with low incomes and very limited assets. These individuals are called qualified medicare beneficiaries (QMBs). Rules vary somewhat from state to state, but the following are general requirements:

1. You must be eligible for Medicare Part A. If you are not eligible for Medicare Part A, Medicaid may buy it for you.

2. Your monthly income must be less than preset limits. These income amounts are adjusted annually; you can obtain the prevailing limits from your area Social Security office.

3. You cannot have resources such as bank accounts, stocks, or bonds worth more than $4,000 for an individual or $6,000 for a couple. Your personal home, auto, furniture, jewelry, life insurance, and burial plot are not counted unless they are of extraordinary value.

For individuals who qualify, Medicaid will cover Medicare premiums, deductibles, and coinsurance costs.

SPECIFIED LOW-INCOME MEDICARE BENEFICIARIES

Individuals who do not qualify for coverage under the qualified medicare beneficiary program because their income is too high may qualify for help under the specified low-income Medicare beneficiary (SLMB) program. There are resource limits, but the monthly income amounts are somewhat higher. Medicaid will pay the Medicare Part B monthly premium for an individual who qualifies. Part B premiums also may be paid for individuals with slightly higher monthly incomes who are qualified individuals (QIs).

More information on both the QMB, SLMB, and QI programs can be obtained by calling your state Medicaid office. For your state Medicaid office phone number refer to the listing in appendix B at the back of this guide.

PARTICIPATING DOCTORS AND SUPPLIERS

Doctors and suppliers who sign agreements to participate in Medicare have agreed in advance to accept assignment on *all* Medicare claims. They may display an emblem in their window that shows they are Medicare participants and thus accept assignment on all Medicare claims. In addition, certain practitioners, such as social workers who provide outpatient mental health services, must accept assignment if they bill Medicare.

Note: All providers, doctors, and suppliers must abide by Medicare laws, even if they choose not to be Medicare

participants. Nonparticipating providers must still provide services to Medicare patients.

Check with your provider or supplier to see if they participate in Medicare or call your carrier (see appendix D) to obtain free of charge the *Medicare Participating Physician/Supplier Directory,* which lists Medicare participants in your area. The directory may also be available to use at your local Social Security office or local hospital.

As mentioned in the section on durable medical equipment (DME), Medicare will pay for claims received *only* from approved suppliers who have a Medicare supplier number.

WHEN PROVIDERS DO NOT ACCEPT ASSIGNMENT

If your doctor or supplier does not accept assignment, you must pay directly. You will usually have to pay the portion of your bill that is greater than the Medicare-approved amount because the provider did *not* agree to accept the Medicare approved amount as payment in full for the item or service. Medicare will pay you 80 percent of the approved amount, less any part of the annual deductible ($100) that you have not met.

Note: *Payment limits* limit the fee any doctor or supplier can charge, even one who does not take assignment. They cannot charge more than 115 percent of the Medicare-approved amount for the service provided; if they do, they are subject to a fine and if you paid more than what the payment limit allows, you may have a refund or reduction in the charge coming to you.

Note: *Elective surgery* is a service with special rules for doctors to follow. They must inform you in advance of the approximate cost of the surgery if it is likely to exceed $500. If the doctor fails to provide you with the written estimate in advance, you are entitled to a refund of any amount you paid over the Medicare-approved amount.

WHO SUBMITS PART B CLAIMS

Doctors, suppliers, and other providers submit claims for Part B services for you, even if they do not accept assignment. Further, they must submit claims within one year or face certain penalties. However, you may need to submit your own claims in certain cases. If you have insurance that should pay *before* Medicare, you should submit those claims yourself. If you must submit your own claim for Part B, be sure to submit it to your regional carrier (see appendix D at the back of this guide). Remember that time frames apply for submission of claims.

If your provider refuses to submit a Part B claim for you for services that you believe are covered by Medicare, notify your Medicare carrier. Part B claims are made by the provider on an HCFA-1550 form. If the claim is for rental or purchase of durable medical equipment, a doctor's prescription or certificate of medical necessity must accompany the claim.

After the claim is submitted, Medicare will send you a notice called "Explanation of Your Medicare Part B Benefits," which will explain the Medicare determination on the claim. The form will list the charges made on the claim and indicate which Medicare approved, what Medicare paid, the copay amount due, and what portion of the deductible, if any, was applied.

CLAIMS FOR DECEASED BENEFICIARIES

When a beneficiary dies, Medicare will pay in a manner dependent on whether the provider's bill has already been paid. If the provider is a hospital, skilled nursing facility, home health agency, or hospice, the Part A claim will be paid directly to the provider as usual. For other services, if the bill was paid by the patient or with funds from the patient's estate, Medicare will make the claim payment to the estate representative or a member of the patient's immediate family. If the bill has been paid by a third party, payment may be made to that individual.

If the bill has not been paid and the provider does not accept assignment, the Medicare payment can be made to the person who has or assumes legal obligation to pay the bill for the deceased.

CARRIERS, INTERMEDIARIES, AND PEER REVIEW ORGANIZATIONS

Carriers are private insurance companies that process Medicare part B claims from doctors and suppliers for the federal government. Claims for durable medical equipment, oxygen, and some other supplies are handled by special carriers called **durable medical equipment regional carriers,** or **DMERCs.** Part B carriers are listed in appendix D at the back of the book; DMERCs are listed in appendix E.

Intermediaries handle inpatient and outpatient claims submitted on your behalf by hospitals, skilled nursing facilities, home health agencies, hospices, and other providers of services under Part A. Generally, any questions you may have concerning Part A can be handled by providers, but they can give you the address and phone number of the regional intermediary that processes their claims if you still have questions. Also, the Notice of Utilization you will receive from Medicare when you use Part A services will identify the intermediary and provide a phone number to call with any questions.

Peer review organizations, or **PROs,** also referred to as quality improvement organizations (QIOs), are groups of doctors and other health care professionals paid by the federal government to review care provided to Medicare recipients. Each state has a peer review organization, which considers whether the care delivered meets applicable standards for quality, whether the care was medically necessary, reasonable, and delivered in an appropriate setting. The PRO can deny payment for the services if it determines that these criteria were not met.

If you are notified by the PRO that payment has been denied, you will also be informed as to whether you are responsible for payment for the services. The addresses and phone numbers for the PROs in each state are listed in appendix F.

The peer review organization in each state also has specific responsibility to address complaints by beneficiaries about the quality of care received. If you feel that the quality of care you received in an acute care hospital, skilled nursing facility, outpatient care facility, emergency room, home health agency, hospice, ambulatory care center, or HMO was poor, you can file a complaint with the PRO for the state in which the organization is located.

The complaint should be in writing, but if you need help in filing a complaint, the PRO will take the information over the phone and write the complaint for you. Further, you may designate someone to speak for you in filing a complaint for the PRO.

REPORTING SUSPECTED FRAUD OR ABUSE OF THE MEDICARE PROGRAM

If you suspect that a doctor, institutional provider (such as a nursing home or home health agency), or supplier of goods (such as home oxygen or durable medical equipment) or other services has provided services that were either unnecessary or inappropriate, or has billed Medicare for services which you did *not* receive, you should report this to the carrier or intermediary that handles your claims.

In August 1996 the Health Insurance Portability and Accountability Act (HIPAA), perhaps better known as the Kennedy-Kassebaum Law, was enacted. This act created some important health insurance protections for consumers and, in addition, created some tough antifraud and anti-abuse provisions. From the consumer's standpoint, a very important aspect of the legislation is found in Section 203, dealing with "whistleblower" protections and incentives for individuals who report suspected fraud or abuse of the Medicare system.

The legislation calls for the creation of rules that will provide financial rewards for individuals who report fraud and abuse, even if it is a past practice and is no longer happening. The actual amount of the reward may be linked to the size of any recovery the government may make against a firm or individual found guilty. The Department of Health and Human Services has set up a fraud reporting hotline number: 1-800-HHS TIPS.

In addition to the Kennedy-Kassebaum provisions just mentioned, there are new penalty provisions in the Balanced Budget Act of 1997. It provides for a civil money penalty

of treble damages plus a $50,000 fine per violation of the Medicare/Medicaid antikickback provisions. The act also provides for permanent exclusion of practitioners and others from participation in the Medicare program if convicted of fraud or abuse. It also allows Medicare not to contract with felons and to exclude from contracts any firms operated by a person related to anyone convicted of fraud.

Another potentially powerful but seldom used law to punish Medicare fraud (and substandard care, for that matter) is the Federal False Claims Act. When used in 1996 against a Pennsylvania nursing home, the government won a $600,000 settlement against the home's owners based on substandard quality of care, which led to decline in the health of several residents, who then required hospitalization. The logic is that the decline was caused by facility's failure to provide adequate care as is required under the Medicare agreement. The facility continued to accept full payment from Medicare but did not deliver all the required care, thus making the facility guilty of filing false claims.

In any case, when calling to report suspected fraud or abuse, be prepared to describe the nature of the problem in some detail, the date it occurred, the name and address of the party involved, the name of your intermediary, and whether you have reported to the intermediary.

■

BALANCED BUDGET ACT BRINGS CHANGES TO THE MEDICARE PROGRAM

A lot of the savings necessary for a claimed balanced budget in the Balanced Budget Act of 1997 came from the Medicare program. The act will cut the growth of spending in the Medicare program from an annual average of 8.5 percent to about 6 percent. In addition to cutting the rate of growth in Medicare spending, the act also changes the formula used for calculating physicians' fees and payments to HMOs and it creates more options for beneficiaries to choose from in terms of the kind of health care delivery system they are in.

The Act created **Medicare+Choice**, also known as **Medicare Part C,** which offers a new set of options for consumers by allowing more types of delivery systems to compete for contracts to administer Medicare benefits. The motivation for this is to encourage more Medicare recipients to participate in managed care plans, which is expected to help generate the savings needed to make the reduction in Medicare spending a reality. In addition, some of the savings realized by the use of managed care may result in plans being able to offer additional benefits such as drug or optical coverage. These benefits may be used to induce people to enroll in managed care organizations.

The act will make it possible for consumers to choose from HMO, point of service (POS), preferred provider organizations (PPOs), provider-sponsored organizations (PSOs), religious fraternal benefit society plans, and private fee-for-service insurance. There also are provisions to allow catastrophic insurance programs that are linked to medical savings accounts. If all of this sounds confusing, it is comforting to know that if you choose not to choose from any of these options, you will still be able to use the more traditional Medicare benefit system.

Provisions for consumers and physicians to contract directly with each other for care also were included in the act. Under **direct contracting,** as it is known, consumers can contract directly with the physician of their choice for their care, but the physician is then obligated to drop out of Medicare participation for two years. Consumers must agree to pay for the service themselves at the rate set by the physician and cannot submit a claim to Medicare for the services provided by the physician.

Medicare beneficiaries need to be aware of the rules and options created by Medicare managed care and should consult with their Social Security Administration benefits specialist for detailed information as well as the managed care entity they plan to enroll in (or "take election," as Medicare rules call it). Enrollment and disenrollment rules from 1998 to 2001 allow the individual to enroll and disenroll with relative ease. However, the rules will change in 2002 and restrictions on enrollment and disenrollment will apply.

The act created some specific requirements that the Health Care Financing Administration (HCFA) is responsible for carrying out. For example, each year, HCFA is required to notify Medicare beneficiaries about

1. The "annual coordinated election period," or open-enrollment period.

2. Benefits available under traditional Medicare, cost sharing, and deductibles.

3. Election procedures for Medicare+Choice.

4. Beneficiary rights information.

5. Information on benefits and rights under Medigap and Medicare Select policies.

6. Available Medicare+Choice plans in the person's area and information about the plans.

7. Quality information on the plans, including data on performance indicators such as disenrollment rates, health outcomes, and member satisfaction survey results.

The act also requires HCFA to conduct a national education program in conjunction with the annual coordinated election period.

Of particular importance to consumers are provisions in the act that deal with grievance and appeal rights, antidiscrimination, denial of enrollment, involuntary disenrollment, disclosure requirements, access to services, provider and practitioner qualifications, out-of-area coverage, quality assurance, accuracy of marketing information, and prohibitions on interference with physician–patient communications. Ask about them if you plan to enroll in managed care.

■

OTHER WAYS TO PAY FOR LONG-TERM CARE

The balance of this chapter is devoted to a discussion of some of the other options that you may wish to use in helping to pay for long-term care. Not all these options are open to everyone. For example, not all areas of the county are served by a Medicare HMO (though that is quickly changing), so this may not be an option, or you may not be able to enroll in a Medicare Select program if it is not available in your state.

MEDIGAP POLICIES

Medicare covers a wide range of health care services and supplies, but there are a number of things it covers only partially or not at all—among them, the cost of long-term care in any facility other than a skilled nursing facility (SNF) or by a home health agency and then only for a limited period of time. This creates some potentially expensive "gaps" in your health insurance protection. To help cover such gaps in Medicare coverage, the law allows companies to sell Medicare supplemental insurance, often referred to as **Medigap insurance.**

Medigap policies must provide specific benefits that pay, within limits, some or all of the cost of services not covered or only partially covered by Medicare. It is important to know that all insurance products designed to cover out-of-pocket health care costs are not necessarily Medigap policies. For example, health plans offered by employers, unions, and some HMOs do not qualify as Medigap policies.

There are 10 standard Medigap policy types, alphabetically designated A through J, specified in the law, and all companies selling Medigap policies must meet the requirements of each type of policy. However, insurers are not required to offer all 10 types of policies; they must make plan A available, but they can decide themselves which of the other nine to offer. The insurer may *not* alter either the combination of benefits in any of the standard plans or the letter designations that apply to each policy type.

Though the law prohibits the insurer from changing the basic content of each of the standard policy types, it does allow the insurer to offer "new and innovative benefits" added to a standard policy that otherwise meets the applicable federal standards. The law requires that any such innovations be "cost effective, not otherwise available in

the marketplace and offered in a manner that is consistent with the goal of simplification."

Medigap policies generally pay the same supplemental benefits regardless of your choice of provider. If Medicare pays for a service, wherever it is provided, the standard Medigap policy must pay its share of the cost. An exception to this is the Medicare Select type of policy.

ELIGIBILITY FOR MEDIGAP COVERAGE

If you are at least 65 years of age, you cannot be denied Medigap insurance or charged higher premiums due to health problems. Open enrollment for Medigap insurance begins on the first day of the effective date of your first enrollment in Medicare Part B and lasts six months from that date. These protections apply if you are 65 or older and enrolling in Medicare for the first time, based on age rather than disability, and if you apply for Medigap within six months of enrollment in Part B.

Even if these conditions are met, "preexisting conditions" may be excluded from coverage for the first six months the policy is in effect. Preexisting conditions are conditions that were either diagnosed or treated during the six-month period before the Medigap policy became effective.

During the six-month open enrollment period, you have the choice of any of the different Medigap policies sold by any insurer doing business in your state. The company cannot deny, delay, or otherwise condition the issuance of a policy on the basis of your medical history, health status, or claims experience. Further, the insurer cannot discriminate in pricing the policy based on any of these factors.

If you are covered under a group health insurance plan through your employer and continue to work past age 65 when you are eligible for Part B, consider your options in light of the fact that once you are enrolled in Medicare Part B, the six-month Medigap enrollment period begins and cannot be repeated or extended. If you are currently enrolled in a Medigap policy that was issued prior to the federal regulations that became effective in 1992, you may not have to switch to a new type of policy, if the policy is guaranteed renewable. Some states, however, may require conversion to a new policy format.

LONG-TERM CARE INSURANCE

In the early 1990s a new option for consumers to use to cover long-term care costs emerged in the marketplace: private long-term care insurance. By 1994, more than 135 companies nationwide were offering private long-term care insurance policies both directly to consumers and through employer groups. While long-term care in a skilled nursing facility or rehabilitation center is covered under Medicare Part A, you must be over 65 to qualify and nearly 40 percent of individuals purchasing long-term care services are under age 65.

Consumers were given some incentive to invest in private long-term care insurance policies for themselves with the passage of the Kennedy-Kassebaum bill. The act makes premiums for long-term care insurance tax deductible, if the individual qualifies. To qualify for the deduction, an individual's health care expenses must exceed 7.5 percent of adjusted gross income.

Another provision of HIPAA may be worth noting, if you are considering some of the creative "estate planning" or "asset protection" services being offered by some financial "experts" and attorneys who claim to specialize in "elder law." The new law provides criminal penalties for anyone who uses such estate planning services to conceal assets so that they may become eligible for Medicaid coverage for their long-term care. The penalties can include a year in jail and fines of up to $10,000. There are many attorneys and financial planners who do provide sound planning services for retirement and investment, so pick a reputable firm or individual and do not be afraid to ask questions. It may be well worth it to consider the investment in purchasing a good long-term care insurance policy instead of trying to qualify for Medicaid.

Long-term care insurance typically covers nursing home care, and some policies cover home health benefits as well.

When you evaluate policies look for whether the following are covered and check on how the policy defines each and what each has for limitations, exclusions, and deductibles. Some of the following tips are based on information from the Health Insurance Association of America (information on how to reach the association appears at the end of this section).[2] Find out if the following types of care are covered:

1. Subacute care.

2. Skilled nursing services (check on what is included in skilled nursing—it may vary).

3. Intermediate nursing services.

4. Custodial or basic nursing services.

5. Alzheimer's disease or dementia care.

6. Therapy services including physical therapy, occupational therapy, respiratory and speech therapy, and psychological/psychiatric care.

7. Medical social worker services.

8. Pharmaceutical benefits.

9. Home health care therapies as listed above which are covered when provided at home or on an outpatient basis.

10. Durable medical equipment.

11. Oxygen therapy and equipment.

12. Coverage of modifications to your home to allow you to remain in your home, such as ramps, grab rails, and bath and kitchen modifications. There may be a maximum benefit amount for this and the use of this benefit may reduce the amount of benefits available for services provided in a nursing home later. Be sure to check the policy's provisions on this.

2. Reprinted with permission of the Health Insurance Association of America.

13. Homemaker, chore services, and other nonnursing services.

If you have private long-term care insurance coverage through an employer group plan as well as Medicare Part A, skilled nursing services would be covered first through the private program and your Medicare coverage would be considered secondary. Since Medicare does not cover care that is considered custodial in nature or that does not require skilled nursing or therapy services (see "Skilled Nursing Care" earlier in this chapter), the private insurance would be of value for covering this type of care.

If you have Medicare Part A and are considering purchasing private long-term care insurance as well, you may be offered the skilled nursing home benefit in the private plan, even though skilled nursing benefits are covered under Part A, such that the private benefit plan would begin paying for skilled nursing *after* the Medicare benefits are exhausted. However, depending on your situation, this may be an expensive option that you never use. Since Medicare pays for the first 20 days of skilled nursing care 100 percent and the next 80 days with a 20 percent copay, a Medigap policy to cover the copay amount may be a better plan. Most people do not require skilled nursing home care for more than 100 days. The most important coverages to consider are those things that Medicare does not cover: custodial long-term care in the nursing home setting, assisted living, or in your home.

As with any insurance coverage, you will want to know about any *exclusions* to the coverage. One common exclusion is coverage for preexisting conditions, which are medical conditions you had when you acquired insurance. Usually, the policy will exclude such conditions from coverage for a set period of time before coverage will be provided. There may be exclusions for coverage of mental illnesses and neurological disorders or substance abuse. In some cases, the policy may require certain preconditions on care. For example, it may require a hospital stay before paying for nursing home care or may require a nursing home stay before coverage is available for home health. Be sure to read the policy thoroughly—remember, what the bold print giveth, the fine print may taketh away.

There are some other conditions or qualifiers that may apply that you need to be aware of. Most policies have age limits: often only those between ages 50 and 85 can purchase a long-term care policy, and the closer your age is to the upper limit of the coverage eligibility range, the more you will pay. The policy will also have a clause that explains its renewability features. Most are guaranteed renewable as long as you pay your premium and the health information you provided on your application was accurate. Look for information in the policy as to when the policy can be canceled or the premiums increased.

The policy will have limits on how long it will pay benefits for various types of care or will set dollar limits for them. Look at the benefit maximums carefully—they vary from one policy to the next and can make a real difference in the value of the policy. For example, a policy may pay up to the maximum benefit in the life of the policy for a given type of care once or it may pay up to a maximum benefit amount for each episode of care.

Ask about a premium waiver feature, which allows you to stop paying the premiums during the time you are collecting benefits. There may be conditions on when this feature applies, if the policy has the feature at all. There may also be provisions in the policy to allow a portion of your premiums paid to be returned to you in the event you drop your coverage, but there may be a cost in terms of higher premiums. This feature is called nonforfeiture.

According to the National Association of Insurance Commissioners, in any long-term care insurance policy, look for the following standards, which are designed to protect you as a consumer:

1. At least one year of nursing home or home health coverage that includes intermediate and custodial care as well as skilled care.

2. Coverage for Alzheimer's disease should the policyholder develop it after purchasing the policy.

3. Inflation protection, usually one of the following: automatic annual initial benefit increases, a guaranteed

right to increase benefit levels periodically without providing evidence of insurability, or covering a specific percentage of actual or reasonable charges.

4. An outline of covered benefits, exclusions, and limitations that makes it easy to compare the policy to others.

5. A shopper's guide that helps you decide if long-term care insurance is right for you.

6. A guarantee that the policy will not be canceled because of age or change of health condition.

7. A right to a premium refund if you decide to cancel the policy within 30 days of its purchase.

8. No requirements for a hospital stay before nursing home or home health benefits can be paid, no requirement that skilled nursing care be provided before intermediate or custodial care benefits can be used, and no requirement that you must receive nursing home care before you can use home health care benefits.

It may be wise to ask about benefits administration. That is, if the policy uses language like "medically reasonable and necessary" or if the policy information indicates that "case management is provided under this policy" in describing what benefits are actually provided under the policy, ask who determines what is "medically reasonable and necessary" and who provides case management. For example, the policy may state that up to 100 days of skilled nursing facility care are covered. However, some insurance companies use another company to do "case management," and the case management firm gets paid to help contain costs. Consequently, such a firm may aggressively work to keep the actual number of days the policy will cover far below what the policy states, based on an assessment of what is medically reasonable and necessary. Thus even the non-HMO insurance policies may, in fact, be administered much like the HMO policies.

For information on long-term care insurance write to the Health Insurance Association of America, 555 13th

Street, NW, Suite 600 East, Washington, DC 20004-1109. You may also call their Insurance Education Program at (202) 824-1673, 1675, or 1852, or visit their website at http://www.hiaa.org.

■

SOURCES OF INFORMATION

Portions of this chapter have been drawn from *The Medicare Handbook 1997*, which your local Social Security Administration office can help you obtain. The Health Care Financing Administration also has a website on the Internet where you can access and download the handbook, other publications, and great information on Medicare. Some of the website addresses that will quickly take you to the information you are likely to find useful are:

HCFA website
http://www.medicare.gov/

Medicare and You
http://www.medicare.gov/publications/handbook.html

Medicare Compare
http://www.medicare.gov/comparison/

1999 Guide to Health Insurance for People with Medicare
http://www.medicare.gov/publications/guide.pdf

Nursing Home Compare
http://www.medicare.gov/nursing/home.asp

Medicare Compare is a site where consumers can obtain information on Medicare HMO plan performance. This can help consumers find out which health plans serve their area and decide which managed care plan to join based on comparison of common performance indicators. Nursing Home Compare is a website added in late 1998. It enables consumers to access information about the most recent surveys of individual nursing homes conducted by state agencies. If you do not own a computer, check out your local public library—they often have computers for public use with Internet connection.

You can also order some federal publications on Medicare. For more information on how Medicare works with other insurance plans and benefits, send for *Medicare and Other Health Benefits,* publication 593B, and the *Guide to Health Insurance for People with Medicare,* publication 518B, available from the Consumer Information Center, Department 33, Pueblo, CO 81009.

3

HMOs

MANAGED CARE IN
LONG-TERM CARE

We cannot leave the subject of paying for care without talking about one of the most important and dizzying changes taking place in health care—the movement toward what is called "managed care." A 1997 study by Louis Harris and Associates, which was reported in *Managed Care* magazine, found that 55 percent of those surveyed were unsure of what "managed care" means. About one-third did not recognize the term "health maintenance organization," and an amazing three-fourths of those surveyed said they never heard of "fee for service" health insurance. I will try to shed some light on these terms and much more about managed care in this chapter.

According to the *Managed Care Digest,* published by Hoechst Marion Roussel, Inc., the number of health maintenance organizations (HMOs) operating in the United States reached 564 by 1994. By that same year, enrollment in HMOs totaled more than 55 million persons, accounting for over 21 percent of the nation's health care market. Medicare recipients in HMOs in 1994 totaled 3.1 million persons; by 1995, the total had grown to 3.6 million.

More and more, states are also channeling their Medicaid recipients into managed care plans in an effort to control costs. In 1994 some 2.7 million Medicaid recipients were covered by HMO plans; by 1995 that number had grown to 4.7 million. Nationwide, HMOs covered 25.7 percent of the nation's health care insurance market in 1995, up from 21.1 percent in 1994. This represents a total of approximately 67.6 million people. All indicators are that despite some controversial issues associated with managed care plans, the number of people insured under them, including those likely to require long-term care, will continue to grow.

One of the most common forms of managed care plan is a health maintenance organization, or HMO. The HMO **prepays** physicians for their members' care, and the organization has case managers who use review criteria called **utilization review guidelines** to decide whether care being proposed is appropriate for the condition being treated. The money paid to physicians is called **capitation.** We discuss this in more detail later in this chapter. Through this process, the HMO attempts to ensure that no unnecessary, excessive, or duplicate services are going to be provided, thus holding costs in check by providing only those services that are medically necessary and reasonable.

There is really nothing new here—Medicare's definition of services that will be covered has always emphasized the mantra "medically necessary and reasonable." The difference is that managed care organizations enforce this requirement by making access to many services and types of care subject to what is known as "prior authorization" or "precertification." Access to speciality care is often subject to approval of a "referral" prior to the first visit to the specialist. These requirements frequently irk both physicians and consumers because they can delay access to care while the prior authorization is being considered, they make it seem as though the insurance company is second-guessing the attending physician, and they often do result in **denials**—the term used to refer to the insurance company's decision not to authorize the requested care.

Health maintenance organizations typically cover most or all of the costs for doctors' office calls, inpatient care, preventive health services such as immunizations, Pap tests, and mammograms, emergency and urgent care, and durable medical equipment. Most plans also have coverage for limited amounts of skilled nursing and home health benefits.

Although the HMO concept is considered to be relatively new, the first HMOs actually started in the 1920s and 1930s in Olkahoma, California, and Oregon. A farmer's cooperative in Elk City, Oklahoma, provided HMO-style health care in the 1920s, and in the 1930s, industrialist Henry Kaiser set up a prepaid health plan for his employees.

The popularity of HMOs continued to grow through the fifties and sixties, despite some strong political opposition. In 1973, Congress passed the Health Maintenance Organization Act. The act encouraged the development of private health care delivery systems like HMOs by doing the following:

1. Preventing state laws from interfering with HMO development.

2. Creating a federal set of qualifying standards.

3. Creating a federal definition of different types of HMOs including group model, staff model, and individual practice association (IPA).

4. Mandating that all employers with more than 25 employees offer HMO health plans if they were available locally.

5. Requiring employers to pay for part of the cost of HMO coverage.

6. Providing funding to help stimulate the growth of HMOs.

Since the passage of the act, HMO (also referred to as managed care organizations, MCOs) membership has grown to the magnitude mentioned at the start of this section. Part of the appeal of the HMO concept is that the HMO is actively involved in coordinating the delivery of care services and takes an interest in health promotion and preventive care as a way to contain costs by keeping members healthy. For care delivered by practitioners either employed by the HMO or under contract with it, the member generally has no claims to file and premiums are generally lower than comparable traditional (referred to as "indemnity" or "fee-for-service") insurance plans.

Because the HMO is, by definition, a system for delivery of health care, it is able to identify resources to provide care and coordinate care among those resources. Because it creates working relationships among the providers and organizations with which it contracts, it can act to contain costs and influence the quality of care its members receive. For the same reasons, it can also be held accountable, at least to some extent, for the costs and quality of care it provides through those providers and organizations.

These characteristics make managed care an appealing option to government agencies and politicians who want to rein in runaway health care costs. A number of mechanisms are used to contain costs in managed care. One is the contracting process: by negotiating discounts and lower fee schedules for services, the HMO can drive down costs for its members. Another tool used to contain costs is utilization management. As mentioned earlier in this chapter, the goal is to identify appropriate care for each case and to avoid duplication and unnecessary tests and procedures. At the federal level, not only has the Medicare program been opened up for managed care contracting, but the Federal Employee Health Benefit Program (FEHBP) and Civilian Health and Medical Program of the Uniformed Services (CHAMPUS, now called Tricare) have as well.

For all the growth and promise of managed care, there is an accompanying set of growing problems. For example, in most managed care plans, members can be treated only by participating (called "par") practitioners or be cared for in participating facilities. Practitioners or facilities are considered to be participating when they have a contract with (or are employed or owned by) the HMO. For many consumers, this presents a roadblock to their ability to choose their own doctor. Also, depending on how many doctors, specialists, and clinics the HMO has available, delays in getting doctors' appointments and long waits at the clinic may be inevitable.

Other problems include instances of needed care being denied or delayed by the lengthy prior authorization processes. In some cases, there have been problems with the requirement for a written referral from the member's primary care physician (PCP), to be approved by the HMO before the member can receive care from a specialist. Since HMOs serve defined geographic areas, there can be problems with getting coverage for care or prescriptions when traveling outside the health plan's defined service area. Though most plans have provisions to cover what they define as true emergencies when the member is out of the plan's service area, other urgent or routine care needs generally will not be covered.

Efforts to cut costs by restricting the length of stay in a hospital have also drawn fire from consumers. One of the most well-known examples of this is the so-called "drive-through delivery," where HMOs limited hospital maternity coverage to one inpatient hospital day. This practice led to so much public indignation that Congress enacted legislation requiring coverage for at least 48 hours of inpatient care following a vaginal delivery and 96 hours of coverage following a cesarian section delivery. Another serious charge

against managed care organizations is that some of them use language in practitioner contracts that would act to limit what the doctor can tell patients about the treatment options open to them, especially if they are of high cost or not available from providers in the plan. Such language is what is known as a "gag clause." There is some dispute about the intent of language in practitioner contracts that may be interpreted as gag clauses, but some states already have legislation prohibiting gag clauses and others are considering it.

The industry is coming under increasing legislative and consumer scrutiny, and there is a growing body of case law arising from civil lawsuits against HMOs for the way some of these problems have contributed to health problems or poor outcomes for their members. At the same time, there is an industrywide movement to improve quality of care and service for individuals served by HMOs.

There are as many as 15 organizations that are providing oversight to the managed care industry by enforcing accreditation standards or by promulgating quality measures for the industry to adopt. There are four we discuss briefly here: the National Committee for Quality Assurance (NCQA), the Joint Commission on Accreditation of Healthcare Organizations (JCAHO), the Utilization Review Accreditation Commission (URAC), which recently changed its name to American Accreditation HealthCare Commission, and FACCT (Foundation for Accountability).

FACCT, which does not engage in accreditation, in late 1996 released a set of proposed managed care performance measures designed to reveal the HMO's performance in key areas. The first five measure sets released include breast cancer, major depressive disorder, diabetes, health risk behavior, and health plan satisfaction.

NCQA has a set of performance measures called HEDIS® 3.0, which was released in 1997. HEDIS® stands for Health Plan Employer Data and Information Set and it includes 75 measures of HMO performance. While the HMO is not required to use HEDIS® for measuring its own performance, many plans are using at least a portion of the measures to track quality improvements. More and more employer groups are requiring performance measures information like HEDIS® as a condition for being considered as the company's insurance carrier and are using this information to compare health plans. Starting in January 1997, HCFA required Medicare managed care plans to report on HEDIS® measures relevant to Medicare enrollees.

NCQA is actively engaged in providing its information both on accreditation status of managed care organizations and on their performance as measured in the HEDIS® report, but HMOs do not all use HEDIS® or seek NCQA accreditation. If you are employed at a company offering a choice of insurance plans at an open-enrollment period, it is likely your employer has already done some comparison shopping among competing companies and may be able to supply information on the health plan's performance. If not, you may be able to get information directly from the insurance company. To learn more about health plans with NCQA accreditation, contact NCQA at 1-(800) 839-6487 or you can access the list on the Internet at http://www.ncqa.org.

NCQA will also supply a copy of the Accreditation Summary Report for any health plan it has reviewed since July 1995. These reports compare how the organization did on the survey to the national averages in specific categories. NCQA also publishes an excellent brochure you may wish to request, *Choosing Quality: Finding the Health Plan That's Right for You.*

IMPLICATIONS OF MANAGED CARE FOR LONG-TERM CARE

Managed care is going to have implications for long-term care providers that may have an impact on the care residents receive. Since the objective of managed care is to achieve genuine cost containment, it's a foregone conclusion that long-term care providers are going to have to make some changes in the way they deliver care. They will have to know their own costs for supplies and labor and manage them precisely on a case-by-case basis. For some facilities, that has been a longstanding practice and the systems for cost tracking and containment are already estab-

lished; for others, especially smaller, individually owned facilities, with less sophisticated management information systems, this may be a new challenge.

The fee-for-service Medicare reimbursement system for long-term care that was in effect prior to the Balanced Budget Act of 1997 had few incentives for cost containment. Indeed, the higher the cost for the care became because of the use of ancillary services such as physical, speech, or occupational therapy, the greater the profit margin could be for the facility. If the costs for Medicare cases were high enough in a facility, the facility could qualify for more reimbursement through what is known as a "routine cost limitation exception." Thus a facility could actually be rewarded for high costs. The Medicare system changed to a prospective payment system (PPS) that will end these problems but may create others (see introduction, p. xviii).

Under managed care, this will not be the case, since these services may be included in a flat rate called a **per diem**, which is negotiated between the HMO and the facility in advance. Excess costs will be the responsibility of the facility, not the patient. In negotiating contracts with HMOs, long-term-care facilities will need to compete with other facilities, since the HMOs will be free to accept the facility offering the most care for the dollar and with the best track record in quality.

WHAT IS CAPITATION?

A reimbursement technique called "capitation" is widely used in managed care. Under capitation, a defined set of services are paid for in advance by the HMO at a rate negotiated with the practitioner or facility providing the services. The capitation amount is usually calculated as a cost to the HMO on a per-member-per-month (PMPM) basis and projected over a period of time, usually a year.

For long-term care providers who are paid under this arrangement, there is what is known as a sharing of "risk" for the financial gain or loss that may result in delivering care. If the capitation rate, or "cap," is too low, or the facility does a poor job managing the cost of care, the facility may lose money. On the other hand, the facility has a strong incentive to manage its costs under the capitation rate, thereby allowing it to profit. This ultimately should be good news for consumers who pay the HMO premiums and taxpayers whose tax dollars support the Medicare fund— as long as access to care and the quality of the necessary services are not compromised in the process.

HMOs can enter the Medicare market under what is called a "risk contract" arrangement with the federal government. Under a Medicare risk contract, the HMO agrees to provide all services the beneficiary would normally receive. The rate of payment the HMO receives is equal to 95 percent of the average cost of care for beneficiaries in a given community. So, the HMO must manage the average cost of its care to be lower than 95 percent of Medicare's average per person expenditure in that area in order to make any money. This is not supposed to affect your quality of care or quality of life in a long-term care facility. The rules governing quality do not change from one payer source to the next. If you have reason to believe they are not being applied equally, discuss the matter with the facility's administration (see chapter 23, "Survey and Enforcement Rules," and appendices I and J).

Managed care organizations like HMOs, unlike the "fiscal intermediaries" who mind the Medicare money in a non-HMO situation, will be very active in the care planning process for their members in long-term care facilities. In some cases this will mean the HMO will send case managers to participate in care planning conferences in the facility. In all cases, it will mean that the HMO will monitor the progress of members in nursing homes quite closely, with the intent to move the member home as soon as possible.

This will tend to shift more cases to home health and community-based care services, which is entirely appropriate in cases where short-term therapy or rehabilitation is required. In cases where *long-term* skilled care is required for recuperation from chronic, severe conditions, there may be times where the interests of the HMO, the long-term care facility, and the individual conflict.

A parallel situation occurred in the 1980s when Medicare introduced the use of diagnosis-related groupings, or DRGs, as a part of a prospective pricing system in its manage-

ment of paying for acute care (hospital) costs. The DRG system is similar to the managed care capitation system in that it places a fixed payment rate on care, but it is different from capitation as practiced in managed care in that it fixes a price for care based on diagnosis, not on a per-member-per-month basis.

The system provides the hospital payment for patient care based on the average cost and length of stay for a given diagnosis. Since the system considers only the *principal* diagnosis, which is the apparent reason for admission, it does not take into account complicating factors that may, under traditional (fee-for-service) payment systems, justify payment for additional hospital days or services. Under prospective pricing, the hospital gets only the amount that is allowed for under the DRG price that applies for that diagnosis, secondary diagnosis, surgical procedure, and age. Once that amount is determined, the hospital must attempt to manage the patient's care to allow the patient to be discharged from the acute care setting before the payment the hospital will receive from Medicare based on the DRG is exceeded.

This has led to the phenomenon of patients under Medicare being discharged "quicker and sicker." The level of complexity of care being required of long-term care facilities and home health agencies is now comparable to care that would have been performed *only* in a hospital setting in the 1980s. There is no reason to expect that Medicare HMOs will be any less aggressive in pushing for discharge from the hospital, but they will also be aggressively pushing for long-term care facility discharge as well.

As managed care principles are applied to long-term care, nursing home stays are generally going to get shorter and care will be more discharge-oriented than ever before. This is not, however, to be accepted by consumers as an excuse for slipshod care, inadequate care, premature or poorly planned discharge, or inappropriate care after discharge.

PAYMENT RULES HAVE CHANGED—QUALITY RULES HAVE NOT

The full sweep of impacts that managed care will have on long-term care is far from being known. The key thing for consumers to remember is that the application of managed care techniques to paying for long-term care does not alter quality of care requirements in OBRA. Likewise, the requirements governing quality of life, residents' rights, and all the other consumer protections apply. Indeed, if you or your loved one is in an HMO, there may be a separate set of rights and protections that apply in addition to those found in OBRA.

By being an informed consumer, family member, or decision maker, you are the most powerful advocate for quality care—do not be afraid to ask a lot of questions, challenge the facility on questionable decisions, insist on complete and accurate information, and demand clear, understandable answers to your questions.

If you have a problem with the care the facility is providing, bring it up first with the facility administration, starting with the director of nursing. If the problem is not resolved at that level, discuss it with the facility administrator. If you are still not satisfied that the problem has been resolved, contact the following agencies.

For quality of care given in the nursing home, contact:

1. The long-term-care ombudsman's office in your state. Their addresses and phone numbers are listed in appendix J at the back of this book.

2. The state survey agency that is responsible for OBRA enforcement for that facility. The phone numbers and addresses are listed in appendix I at the back of this book.

For quality of care provided by your doctor, contact:

The Medicare PRO (or QIO) in your state (listed in appendix F).

For problems with insurance coverage such as denial of care, involuntary disenrollment, excessive premiums, or suspected fraud:

1. Call your HMO's customer service number.

2. Call the free insurance information and counseling line in your state. They are listed in appendix C.

3. Write to: Office of Managed Care, Room 4406, Cohen Building, 330 Independence Avenue, SW, Washington, DC 20201.

4. Contact your state office of the commissioner of insurance listed in appendix M.

TERMS USED IN MANAGED CARE

ACCESS
A patient's ability to reach the physician by phone, the ability to make appointments for care, the length of time in the waiting room before seeing the physician. This term can also be used to refer to the geographic availability of primary and specialty care providers and facilities.

AFTERCARE
Services that are provided as the next step in the person's recuperation after services delivered in the hospital or nursing home.

AMBULATORY CARE
Care given in a clinic or specialized setting that the patient comes to and departs from the same day. Also called **outpatient care.**

ANCILLARY SERVICES
Physical therapy, speech therapy, respiratory therapy, occupational therapy, radiology, lab services, and the like.

AUTHORIZATION

Insurance company or government payer source (e.g., Medicaid) approval, which must be obtained before a service can be rendered and paid for. Also termed **certification** or **prior authorization.**

BOARD CERTIFICATION

Attestation that a physician has successfully completed a medical specialty board's examination.

BOARD ELIGIBILITY

Denotation that a physician has completed the required training in a medical specialty area and is eligible to take that specialty board's examination.

CAPITATION

The practice in managed care of paying a fixed amount to a provider or entity to cover the cost of providing care to members of a health plan for a set period of time.

CARVE OUT

An arrangement whereby certain services are provided and managed by an entity other than the HMO.

CASE MANAGEMENT

The process of deciding which services are necessary and appropriate for a given case and ensuring that they are available and used as needed so that no unnecessary costs are added to the case.

CERTIFICATION

See AUTHORIZATION.

CHEMICALLY EQUIVALENT MEDICATIONS

Generic medications used to take the place of brand-name medications. Generic medications are frequently used in restricted or closed formularies in managed care as a way of holding down the cost of medications.

CLOSED FORMULARY

Limited range of medications covered through the health plan. Managed care plans limit available medications to encourage the use of generic or specific types of medications.

COINSURANCE

The percentage of the cost of care that is paid by the consumer. Also referred to as a **copayment.**

CONCURRENT REVIEW

Evaluation of care or treatment being provided as it progresses, for example, the review that is conducted on hospital care while the member is still in the hospital.

COST-BASED REIMBURSEMENT

Payment to providers based on the actual cost of care.

CREDENTIALING

An approval process used by managed care organizations, hospitals, and other medical organizations to ensure that the practitioners that they employ or contract with are qualified by training, licensure, and experience to perform the care required.

DEDUCTIBLE

A fixed amount that the consumer is expected to pay in a fixed time period before the insurance begins to pay for care. For example, a $500 deductible means that the first $500 of care is paid for by the consumer, generally within a year, before the insurance coverage begins to pay.

DURABLE MEDICAL EQUIPMENT (DME)

Walkers, wheelchairs, canes, bathroom grab rails, shower chairs, lift chairs, hospital beds, oxygen equipment, and other reusable medical equipment.

ENROLLMENT

The process of joining an HMO. This term is also used to refer to the total HMO membership.

EPISODE OF CARE

The entire course of treatment for a specific period of illness.

EXCLUSIVE PROVIDER ORGANIZATION (EPO)

An arrangement which requires members receive care only from participating providers in the organization to receive full coverage for the cost of care.

FEDERALLY QUALIFIED HMO (FQHMO)

A health maintenance organization that meets the requirements of the HMO Act of 1973 and its amendments.

FEE FOR SERVICE

The traditional method of payment to providers for care provided based on fees set by the provider.

FEE SCHEDULE

A preset schedule of rates paid to providers by the insurer for specific services.

FORMULARY

A frequently revised listing of medications available to plan members. *See also* CLOSED FORMULARY.

GATEKEEPER

The role usually assumed by a person's primary care doctor in an HMO plan to coordinate the person's care and use of ancillary and specialty services. By this mechanism, the primary care physician becomes an important part of the cost control system for care as well.

GRIEVANCE PROCEDURE

The set of steps the member and the HMO must follow to address member concerns or dissatisfaction. Some elements of the procedure are dictated by state law.

GROUP MODEL HMO

An arrangement where the HMO contracts with physician group practice(s) for the provision of care to the HMO's members.

HEDIS ®

Health Plan Employer Data and Information Set, a set of performance measures developed by the National Committee for Quality Assurance (NCQA) to help employers and consumers evaluate and compare the performance of one health plan with another.

HOME HEALTH CARE

The delivery of health care services—complex skilled nursing, personal care, physical therapy, occupational therapy, social services, and so on—in the patient's home.

HYBRID MODEL HMO

The combination of more than one type of HMO to form a single managed care organization.

INDEMNITY PLAN

Coverage in which health services are paid for on a fee-for-service basis.

INDIVIDUAL PRACTICE ASSOCIATION (IPA)

An arrangement where the HMO contracts with a physician organization, which, in turn, has contracts with individual physicians. The physicians may see members of other health plans and fee-for-service patients as well. The HMO pays the IPA and the IPA then pays the physicians.

LENGTH OF STAY (LOS)
The number of consecutive days a person is in a hospital or long-term-care facility for a given episode of care.

MANAGED CARE ORGANIZATION (MCO)
A health insurance plan under which the insurance company plays a role in managing the delivery of care in order to control costs. HMOs are examples of managed care organizations.

NETWORK
The group of providers and facilities linked by contractual agreements to a managed care organization to provide care to its members. This may include physicians and other clinicians, hospitals, clinics, nursing homes, therapists, pharmacists, counselors, home health agencies, and laboratories.

OUT OF POCKET (OOP)
Costs that must be paid by the consumer. The abbreviation OOP also can refer to care received "out of plan," or outside the network of providers that make up a managed care organization's network. This care usually will not be covered by the HMO unless the member has what is known as a "point-of-service" plan or substantial copay amounts will apply.

PEER REVIEW
A process by which practitioners evaluate the quality and appropriateness of care provided by a facility or other practitioner.

PHYSICIAN–HOSPITAL ORGANIZATION (PHO)
An arrangement where a hospital and its physicians are mutually committed to payer contracts.

POINT OF SERVICE (POS)
A managed care plan option that allows the member to go to any provider, even out of the plan's service area, but applies copays to such care.

PREFERRED PROVIDER ORGANIZATION (PPO)
A managed care arrangement that allows members to use providers that are not in the PPO network but provides financial incentives to use network providers.

PRIMARY CARE PHYSICIAN (PCP)
The physician whom the HMO member has selected to be his or her principal doctor. The PCP renders most care, makes decisions about hospital care, and makes decisions about referrals to specialists.

PRIOR AUTHORIZATION
See AUTHORIZATION.

PROVIDER
A practitioner or facility rendering care. In some cases, the term *practitioner* refers only to a physician or other caregiver and the term *provider* refers only to institutional entities such as hospitals, nursing homes, and home health agencies.

QUALITY ASSURANCE (QA), QUALITY IMPROVEMENT (QI), CONTINUOUS QUALITY IMPROVEMENT (CQI)
Processes and systems used to ensure conformity to standards of quality, identify problems, and improve on quality of care and services.

SECONDARY CARE
Required care beyond that which the PCP can provide in the local clinic; generally provided by a specialist.

STAFF MODEL HMO
Managed care plan in which the physicians and other clinical staff are employees of the HMO.

TERTIARY CARE

Highly specialized care, generally requiring the use of a facility that delivers specialty care. Sometimes referred to as **subspecialty care.**

TRIAGE

Sorting and prioritizing the delivery of care based on the severity of injury or illness.

URGENT CARE

Nonemergency care that is required in a relatively short period of time. Some HMOs operate urgent care centers for use by members whose situation will not allow them to wait until a clinic appointment is available but who do not require the use of a much more expensive hospital emergency room.

UTILIZATION REVIEW

A process for evaluation of the necessity and cost-effectiveness of clinical services and facilities.

4

Alzheimer's Disease

According to statistics from the National Institutes of Health, dementia in America's adult population is a major and growing medical and social problem. The occurrence of dementing illnesses is the highest in the population over age 75. This is also the age group that is growing in number at a higher rate than any other, according to the U.S. Bureau of the Census. Thus dementia is a frequent diagnosis among nursing home residents.

Dementia is a condition that is poorly understood. Even if you have the clinical definition in writing, it can be difficult to grasp. Here is the clinical definition of dementia:

A clinical state with many different causes, characterized by a decline from a previously attained intellectual level. The decline usually involves memory, other cognitive capacities, and adaptive behavior. There is usually no major alteration of consciousness. The patient may or may not be aware of the dementia. In most cases, there is significant deterioration of memory and one or more other intellectual functions such as language, spatial or temporal orientation, judgment, and abstract thought. Some criteria for dementia require defects in one or more components in intellectual function other than memory; some require that the defect be global, that is involve all components of intellectual function. Dementia is a consequence of dysfunction of the brain, particularly those parts of the cerebrum known collectively as the association areas, which integrate perception, thought, and purposeful action so that the person can adjust to and survive in the environment.[1]

That lengthy definition applies to two types of cognitive impairments: those that are temporary and can be reversed and those that are chronic and irreversible. There are a number of treatable conditions which can cause symptoms that are identical to the symptoms of the chronic, irreversible disease processes that cause dementia. For this reason, when symptoms of apparent dementia occur, it is vital that a thorough physical examination be done by a doctor to determine the cause of the symptoms. The following conditions can cause symptoms that *resemble* dementia but are actually *treatable* symptoms of a temporary condition known as delirium:

1. Nutritional disorders and deficiencies.

2. Dehydration.

1. "Differential Diagnosis of Dementing Diseases," *NIH Consensus Development Conference Statement* 6, no. 11, July 1987.

3. Renal (kidney) failure.

4. Thyroid disease.

5. Pulmonary (lung) disease.

6. Cardiovascular (heart and vessel) disease.

7. Infections.

8. Drug toxicities, interactions, or reactions.

9. Brain tumor.

10. Affective disorder.

11. Depression (left untreated, depression is associated with increased risk for the development of dementia).

The most common causes of permanent or irreversible dementia are progressive degenerative diseases, including:

1. Alzheimer's disease.

2. Lewy body dementia.

3. Amyotrophic lateral sclerosis (ALS), commonly referred to as Lou Gehrig's disease.

4. Huntington's chorea (also referred to as Huntington's disease).

5. Olivopontocerebellar atrophy.

6. Parkinson's disease.

7. Pick's disease (also known as Pick's atrophy).

Of these, by far the most common is Alzheimer's disease, which is believed to account for 55 percent of all dementia cases. Nationwide, it is estimated that more than 4 million people have Alzheimer's disease. It has been estimated that by the year 2050, as many as 14 million people could be affected.

Alzheimer's disease is named for Dr. Alois Alzheimer, a German psychiatrist who first described the neural changes that occur in the brain of Alzheimer's disease patients in 1907. The neural changes he described are neuritic plaques and nerve fiber tangles that have come to be known as the characteristic abnormal brain changes caused by Alzheimer's disease. The disease affects parts of the brain that control thought, memory, language, attention, and judgment.

■

THE SIGNS AND SYMPTOMS OF ALZHEIMER'S DISEASE

The signs and symptoms of Alzheimer's disease affect both mental and physical functioning. The nerve tissue in the brain develops the plaques and tangles that Alzheimer described, which are considered the key *physical* diagnostic feature of the disease. Unfortunately, that diagnostic feature can be determined only by brain tissue biopsy after the patient has died. Other diagnostic indicators do exist, but no single diagnostic test is considered to be completely accurate in establishing the diagnosis of Alzheimer's disease.

An accurate diagnosis depends on the use of a detailed history of symptoms, lab work, and a thorough physical examination by the physician to rule out other causes. A recent development is the use of a blood test to look for levels of a substance known as amyloid protein, which is considered a highly accurate indicator for the presence of the disease, but the use of the test is still being studied. The following listing covers the most common signs of Alzheimer's disease.

EARLY SIGNS

1. Gradual memory loss and confusion.

2. Communication difficulties.

3. Impaired problem solving and reasoning.

4. Disorientation in familiar places.

5. Mood swings or bursts of anger.

6. Changes in personality.

7. Suspicion.

8. Loss of initiative.

LATER SIGNS

1. Stammering, stuttering, or garbled speech.

2. Aimless wandering.

3. Unawareness of personal danger.

4. Agitated or physically aggressive behavior.

5. Severe and eventually total debilitation. Ultimately, the disease is fatal.

Intensive research on Alzheimer's disease is being conducted at 17 divisions of the National Institutes of Health and through nearly 30 Alzheimer's Disease Centers (ADCs) at major medical centers across the country. Although the causes of the disease are still unknown and there is no cure, the Food and Drug Administration has approved new medications for use in treating the symptoms of the disease. For the foreseeable future, however, care for the Alzheimer's disease patient will center on maintaining existing functions for as long as possible, providing emotional support, ensuring safety, promoting optimal health, and providing support for the family.

In the early stages of the disease, caring for the individual at home may be accomplished by family members. Assistance by home health providers, local agencies that provide home and community-based support services, and guidance from the physician can facilitate care at home. As the disease progresses, the care needs of the patient may become so challenging that the family caregivers are overwhelmed, even with the support of outside agencies. Behavioral changes such as aggression, agitation, and suspicion as well as safety issues such as wandering and falls and the increasing need for assistance with eating, bathing, dressing, and grooming may eventually make it impossible to meet the individual's care needs at home.

When family members are caregivers for a person with Alzheimer's disease, even with supportive services being provided, it is vital that they establish links to community support groups and make an effort to care for themselves. This is particularly true for an elderly spouse or other older family members. There is evidence of a relatively high mortality rate among family caregivers for Alzheimer's disease patients.

■

DEMENTIA CARE IN A FACILITY SETTING

Although most individuals with Alzheimer's disease who are placed in a nursing home are likely to be placed in a facility that does *not* have any type of separate wing or unit for dementia patients, the number of facilities that feature dementia specialized care units is growing (see figure 3). Further, the number of facilities that are custom-built specifically for the care of individuals with dementia is also growing.

A lot of research has been done on how to design facilities and treatment programs to meet the needs of dementia patients and their families, yet there is still much to learn. Not all experts agree on the characteristics those programs and facilities should have, but some common characteristics have been identified in recent studies:

1. Admission criteria restrict admission to individuals suffering with symptoms of dementia.

2. Staff receive specialized training in the care of patients with dementia.

3. The activities program is specifically designed for individuals with cognitive impairments.

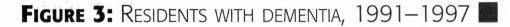

FIGURE 3: RESIDENTS WITH DEMENTIA, 1991–1997

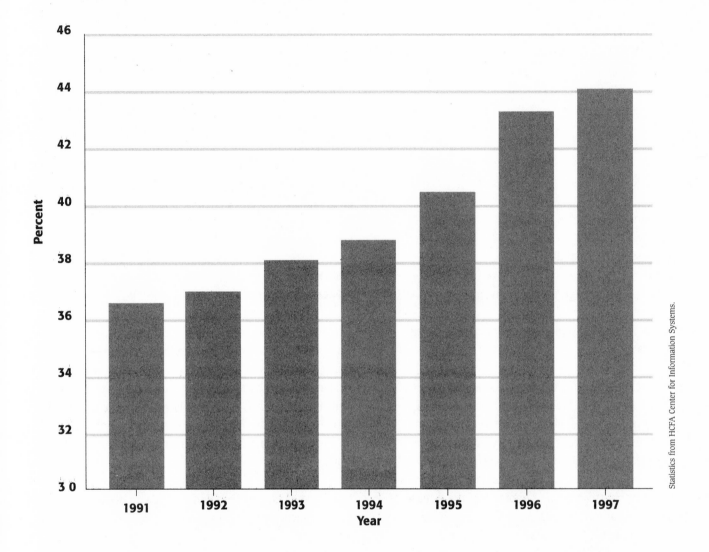

Statistics from HCFA Center for Information Systems.

The prevalence of a diagnosis of dementia among nursing home residents is climbing rapidly. In 1991, some 36.6 percent of the nation's nursing home residents were reported to have a diagnosis of dementia. By 1997, that number had risen to 44.1 percent. This trend coupled with a rising trend of residents with psychiatric diagnoses may be factors in the dramatic increase in the use of psychoactive drugs in the nation's nursing homes.

4. The specialized care unit is separate and has its own director.

5. Family involvement is encouraged.

6. The physical environment is designed to promote both safety and independence; it is homelike and allows the resident to wander at will with supervised safety.

7. The interior design avoids hard, glossy tile floors in favor of low-loop carpeting.

8. Indirect, shadow-free lighting is used to prevent glare, which can be a source of sensory stimulation that can lead to agitated behavior or visual difficulty.

9. Furnishings are residential in type, not institutional, with styles that do not have sharp edges or corners.

10. Pictogram signage or color coding and open floor plan design help the resident navigate independently.

11. Facility design avoids the use of stairs.

12. The environment and operations minimize noise.

13. Behavioral health services such as family therapy and counseling are available.

14. Policies on the use and monitoring of psychoactive medications are comprehensive.

15. The facility is equipped with wanderer protection security systems.

16. Policies on the use of restraints—monitoring, reduction, and alternatives—are comprehensive.

17. Dietary and nutritional risk (weight loss prevention) policies and programs are used.

18. Family education programs and reference materials are available and there is a support group on site or affiliated.

For additional information resources dealing with Alzheimer's disease, see appendix H.

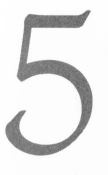

5

Choosing a Long-Term Care Facility

It Is Not Just a Building

Once you know who pays for what, how do you find the facility that meets your needs? Handy checklists on choosing a long-term care facility frequently recommend that you start by touring local nursing homes. That may sound like commonsense advice—the building *is* important and you can tell *some* things about a facility by how it looks. But there are more important things that should be considered first in selecting a facility.

Begin the search at home: look at the care needs of the person for whom the long-term care placement is being arranged. What are the current care needs and what do you anticipate them to be by the time of admission? The most important aspect of finding the right long-term care facility is to first find one that is both licensed for and capable of delivering the types of care and therapy that are needed.

For example, if the facility is to be used for recovery and rehabilitation after an elective orthopedic surgery such as a hip or knee replacement, a facility with physical therapy capability will be necessary, preferably available at least five days a week. There may be the need for occupational therapy and respiratory therapy as well, depending on what other health conditions the person is coping with. In basic nursing homes, referred to as nursing facilities (NFs) in technical jargon, such therapies are not available, so in this case touring NFs would be a waste of time.

If an individual needs care for Alzheimer's disease or other forms of dementia, it would be wise to look for a facility that specializes in that type of care, either facilitywide or as a number of facilities have available, in what is called a specialized care unit, or SCU, as discussed in chapter 4. A word of caution here: if the facility says it has a specialized care unit, ask for a detailed description of how the care and staffing patterns in that unit differ from the rest of the facility. This is the only way to get an idea of whether and to what extent the care is really specialized. Other facilities do not have dementia units but do admit individuals suffering with dementia. In those facilities, find out how they meet the distinct needs of people with dementia and how they train their staff to take care of them.

The point is, identify the key care needs to be met and try to identify the facilities that are capable of meeting those needs. How can this be done? First, invite your doctor's opinion—generally doctors know which facilities do what in their practice area. The yellow pages listings in your phone book may have ads with information on the types of care facilities can provide. If the advertisement does not say what care the facility provides, the facility will generally give you the information you need by phone. Finally, you may be able to get information from your state's agency on aging (see appendix G).

Once you have identified some appropriate options, do a little research on the facilities in terms of quality of care. Your physician may be able to make a recommendation on this topic as well. Another source of information on this topic may be the state long-term care ombudsman's office (see appendix J) or the state survey agency (see appendix I). These agencies may be able to provide specific survey information on the facility's history of deficiencies and whether there have been any allegations or complaint surveys or visits against the facility. If you are planning far enough ahead, you can request a copy of the survey reports for the facilities you are considering from the state survey agency. The reports are available to the public, but you should expect to pay a copying fee if you request copies. After obtaining copies of survey reports you can compare competing facilities and, should you tour a facility, you can take the survey report with you and ask any questions about issues identified in the survey, particularly about how the facility has corrected the deficiencies. You may also obtain survey information at HCFA's Nursing Home Compare website on the Internet at http://www.medicare.gov/nursing/home.asp.

Members of the local senior citizens group may also have information or be able to refer you to individuals with experience with a given facility. Another good source of information about long-term care facilities is the hospital discharge planning or social services staff.

When you are discussing these placement issues, verify that the physician of your choice has admitting privileges at the facilities being considered. It would be dismaying to find what appears to be the best facility only to discover that the physician of your choice does not see patients in the facility. If you belong to an HMO or other managed care organiza-tion, your care will be linked to a facility that has a contract with that organization, so ask your HMO for information on which facilities are available to you. In addition, many managed care organizations conduct their own quality-of-care assessments for long-term care facilities, so they may be a good source of information as well.

Unfortunately, 68 percent of all admissions to nursing facilities and skilled nursing facilities take place directly after discharge from an acute care hospital. Most often this happens when the hospitalization was necessitated by a sudden medical event like a stroke or a serious injury. This situation requires that many issues be resolved in a very short period of time. Shopping for a long-term care facility in a way that allows all the important factors to be considered may be impossible. One way to help offset this problem is to begin discussing long-term care placement options with the hospital discharge planners as soon as it becomes evident that nursing home placement will be necessary. For the patient, this may be very difficult; for a family member or decision maker, it can allow at least some time to do a little comparison shopping before the hospital discharge date arrives.

In many cases discharge to a nursing home is not the only option, even if significant nursing and therapy needs have to be met. Home health agencies are able to do a great deal of care that only a few years ago would have been done only in an inpatient setting. The viability of home health nursing is greatly enhanced when a spouse or family member can be at home with the person being discharged. Another option becoming more common these days is the assisted living facility.

If the hospital discharge plan does require a nursing facility or skilled nursing facility, or you are doing some advance planning for an elective admission, it will be helpful to have a tool to use for identifying facilities that may be able to provide the care required and for making comparisons among facilities. Appendix P is a selection planner for long-term care to assist consumers with this difficult but important decision.

Home, Safe Home

REQUIREMENTS FOR A SAFE,
HOMELIKE ENVIRONMENT

Over the years, I have visited facilities so clean, fresh-smelling, even elegant that I felt like moving in myself. These facilities stand as a tribute to the people who designed and built them, as well as to the staff and administrators who keep them that way every day. Sadly, I have also seen facilities that "smell like a nursing home" and "look like a nursing home." Many readers will know what I mean by that. The well-worn traditional view of a nursing home has been shaped by facilities that

1. Have a persistent odor of urine, feces, or strong disinfectants.

2. Have rooms and hallways that are dingy, dim, and uninviting.

3. Have dark, beaten woodwork, if any, and floor surfaces covered in worn, hard tile.

4. Have few wall hangings, artwork, or decorative accents.

5. Have dull or dingy wall coverings.

6. Have small, old, and dingy windows.

7. Have furnishings that are old, mismatched, and in poor repair.

8. Have plumbing fixtures that are old and in poor repair.

9. Have inefficient, drafty heating systems, which leave cold spots or whole rooms colder than others, and have no air conditioning or limit it to certain areas.

10. Have an "institutional" feeling, more akin to a hospital ward than a homelike environment.

11. Have poorly maintained building exteriors and grounds that are not equipped to encourage outdoor activities by residents.

I have seen facilities that have many of these characteristics. Fortunately, there are a growing number of facilities that look more like this:

1. The air in the building is fresh or pleasantly scented, and it is well-ventilated throughout.

2. Hallways and living and dining areas are well lighted yet free of glare.

3. All areas are attractively decorated and inviting, with wall coverings in warm colors and attractive textures and patterns.

4. Hallways, rooms, and living areas are kept free of hampers, linen carts, and clutter.

5. Furniture is new, comfortable, and in good repair, fit for a home, not a town hall.

6. Floor coverings are in good repair and include carpeting in living areas.

7. Amenities include attractive curtains, window treatments, wall decorations, and living area accessories.

8. Woodwork and cabinetry are in good repair.

9. The facility is clean.

10. Heating and cooling equipment and plumbing are modern and in good repair.

11. If not fully air-conditioned, the facility has common areas that are.

12. The grounds are clean and equipped with benches, tables, and recreational areas for outdoor activities, and the exterior of the building is well-maintained.

Notice that age is not mentioned in the preceding list. With thoughtful design, old buildings can have charm and character while being attractive and functional as well.

Now that we have covered characteristics not mandated in OBRA that can help you define whether the facility's environment is not only safe but homelike and pleasant to live in, we will go on to things that are covered in the rules.

■

SAFETY AND COMFORT

In facilities that house a large number of people, safety—particularly fire safety—is always a concern. The standards that apply are drawn from other sets of regulations called life safety codes that are not part of OBRA but apply to long-term care facilities. The principal code which applies is the Life Safety Code of the National Fire Protection Association. This code deals with issues such as the number of fire exits the building must have, where they must be located, rules about fire exit accessibility, fire alarm and fire suppression systems, and building construction details that bear on the issue of fire safety. (References on this part of the OBRA rules are in 42 CFR Sec. 483.70(a).)

Inspection of long-term care facilities for compliance may actually cross jurisdictions, with local fire departments conducting periodic inspections and the state also providing inspection on an annual basis. Their reports should be available for your examination. The state report will be available as well since it is made a part of the facility's state survey report, even though the two inspections may not occur together.

Ask to see the facility's *fire and disaster plan* if it is not provided during the admission process. This is a written plan that describes how the facility responds to a fire in the facility, flooding, tornado or hurricane threats, gas leak emergencies, utility failures (e.g., power outages and loss of water supply), bomb threats, and the like. Do not expect to see much detail about bomb threat procedures, since some aspects of those plans work best if they are not known to the general public.

In addition to requirements that deal with fire safety, the regulations also provide requirements that cover the physical plant (the building itself). The facility is required to have an emergency electrical power generation system that is sufficient in capacity to provide lighting at all of the exits. For facilities that use life support systems (mechanical ventilators), the facility must have a generator system that starts automatically within 10 seconds of a power failure.

There are specific requirements for the amount of floor space in each resident room. Semiprivate rooms, which accommodate more than one resident, must contain at least 80 square feet of floor space per resident; private rooms, which accommodate one resident, must be at least 100 square feet. Rooms may not be designed to house more than four residents and must be designed and equipped to allow for adequate nursing care, comfort, and privacy for the residents. The facility may get a waiver for smaller room sizes if the building was constructed before the floor space requirements took effect.

Each resident room must be equipped to provide for visual privacy. That means there must be equipment such as ceiling-to-floor cubicle curtains or movable screens to allow privacy during care such as bathing and dressing while the person's roommate is still in the room. The most important aspect of personal privacy is usually not the presence or absence of the equipment—the presence of the equipment is ensured by the survey process—but the actual *use* of the privacy equipment that is available.

Resident rooms must have a window that opens to the exterior of the building or to an atrium. This requirement has both fire safety and quality-of-life implications since it allows natural light into the living space, can facilitate movement of fresh air into the room, and can help the resident maintain orientation to surroundings, location, and time of day.

All of the rooms must be at or above grade (ground) level. This means that the facility cannot convert any basement space into living space for its resident population unless the foundation is excavated and the room meets the window requirement.

The facility must equip each room with a bed and functional furnishings appropriate to the needs of each resident in the room. The bed's mattress must be clean and comfortable and bedding must be clean and appropriate to the climate the facility is in. The choice of mattress can be a serious problem at times. Because institutional-style mattresses, such as those used for hospital beds, tend to be quite firm, which does not suit every resident, ensuring the comfort of residents can be difficult, even if mattresses are changed.

The use of what is called an "eggcrate," or convoluted foam mattress overlay, can help improve the situation in some cases.

"Functional furnishings" is a term that would seem to have obvious meaning, but its interpretation varies under different circumstances. OBRA requires that

> *the furniture in each resident's room contributes to the resident attaining or maintaining his or her highest practicable level of independence and well-being.*
>
> *[42 CFR Sec. 483.70(d)(2)(iv)]*

What this means in practical terms, for example, is that if a resident's room is equipped with chairs that have seating height so low that it inhibits the resident's ability to stand up independently from sitting in the chair, then the facility should arrange for a chair with seating height that allows the resident to rise unassisted to be placed in the room. This will enable the resident who has this physical capability to maintain the highest level of independent mobility.

The same rule could apply to chairs with or without armrests. If a chair with armrests enables the resident to rise to a standing position without requiring staff assistance, then a chair with armrests should be offered among that resident's room furnishings.

To the greatest extent possible, closet space should be accessible to residents. Drawers should also be accessible, and commonly used items or possessions should be within easy reach.

Lighting in a facility is not only a powerful element in how the facility appears when consumers tour the building, but it also has real importance in the residents' quality of life and safety. The lighting and colors in the facility can make it seem cold, drab, or institutional; or, when carefully planned, they can make the facility appear warm and inviting. The use of diffuse, reflected lighting instead of bright, direct lighting can make the facility bright but prevent glare, shadows, and dark corners.

For facilities that care for residents with Alzheimer's disease, this type of lighting can have therapeutic value. Bright, glaring lights tend to be particularly troublesome for individuals with Alzheimer's disease, in some cases thought to contribute to agitated or aggressive behavior. Diffuse lighting that is softened by reflection off the ceiling or alcove tends to benefit the dementia patient by reducing shadows, which may be misinterpreted as objects, holes, or steps and can increase the risk of falls.

In some states, light levels are actually prescribed by rule and enforced by direct measurement using a lightmeter. The drawback to this system is that it measures only light levels, not how well the lighting is delivered. Other states look at the issue from a design standpoint, evaluating the engineering plans for watts per square foot of floor space. This is even more incomprehensible from the consumer's point of view and also does not consider the problems of glare and shadow. The OBRA standard for lighting probably makes the most sense from a consumer's point of view, though it is subjective and therefore hard to enforce. It simply mandates

> *adequate and comfortable lighting levels in all areas.*
>
> *[42 CFR Sec. 483.15(h)(5)]*

The term "adequate lighting" is defined as levels of illumination "suitable to tasks the resident chooses to perform or the facility staff must perform."

HOUSEKEEPING AND MAINTENANCE

In some facilities, housekeeping and maintenance functions are combined in one department, which may also include the in-house laundry if the facility provides laundry services. These functions may also be termed "environmental services." How these functions are organized in a given facility is less important from the consumer standpoint than how well they perform.

Keeping the facility clean and orderly is essential to providing an environment that is safe and healthy for residents to live in. A clean, orderly environment does more than just look good. It contributes to the residents' sense of well-being, to fall prevention, to comfort, and to infection control. How meticulous a facility's administration is about the cleanliness and functionality of the resident's living environment is one indicator of how meticulous the facility is about all aspects of care.

Nursing homes in the past had a reputation for "smelling like a nursing home." Odors from urine or feces make for an unpleasant living experience. Although the presence of these odors in the long-term care facility is inevitable, they need not be constant and pervasive in the building. If the facility ensures that staff are available, trained, and equipped to clean commodes, bedpans, soiled linens, and spills quickly, these odors can be virtually eliminated. The use of air-freshening agents and adequate building ventilation can help keep the living space fresh and pleasant.

In addition to sniffing around, look for clean floors, draperies, window glass, furniture, wheelchairs, and tabletops and orderly living and activity areas to get a feel for how well the facility handles the housekeeping functions on a day-to-day basis.

How well the facility is maintained can be apparent, but what you can see may not tell the whole story. For example, the maintenance staff may oversee the building's internal communications systems, fire alarm, and security systems and may be responsible for most maintenance and testing of the facility's fire suppression or sprinkler system, if the facility is so equipped.

Consumers may wish to ask what fire safety systems are in place and who maintains them as well as who maintains the fire extinguishers in the facility. A very good question to ask of facility staff that bears directly on the preparedness of the facility to handle an emergency is how often the facility has fire drills on each shift. The facility should keep a fire drill log, so if you ask a staff member what he or she is supposed to do when the fire alarm goes off and that staff member does not know, you may wish to ask the facility about this in more detail.

The facility's heating and cooling systems may also be the responsibility of the maintenance staff. The standards in 42 CFR Sec. 483.15(h)(6) require that the temperature in the facility be between 71 and 81 degrees year-round. Though facilities certified before October 1, 1990, do not necessarily have to comply with this specific range, they all must stay in a "comfortable" range, which is not likely to be allowed to stray from the stated range for too long a period. During a summer heat wave, for example, facilities may be allowed to exceed the 81 degree mark, but the facility is then responsible to take actions to keep the residents from suffering ill effects from the heat by supplying fans, ventilation, and extra fluids as needed. Likewise, if the facility for any reason cannot avoid going below the minimum temperature, the facility must take measures to compensate.

More easily assessed items to look for that reflect the attitudes of the facility's administration toward maintenance include the upkeep and appearance of the building's exterior and grounds, condition of the woodwork, doors, privacy curtains, in-room furniture, plumbing fixtures, and lights.

Laundry services, whether in-house or contracted to others, must provide an adequate supply of clean bath linens, bed linens, and clothing to the facility's residents each day, weekends included. That is a big job, even in a small facility.

■

DIETARY SERVICES

The implications of the success or failure of the facility's dietary services are very significant in the quality of care and the quality of life enjoyed or endured by residents. Let's face it—for a great many people, nothing beats a good meal and if the facility fails to deliver it, everything else in the day, however well done, will be diminished.

This fact is not lost on the framers of the OBRA legislation. Dietary services are therefore regulated from several perspectives in the regulations. The requirements for dietary services state:

The facility must provide each resident with a nourishing, palatable, well-balanced diet that meets the daily nutritional and special dietary needs of each resident.

[42 CFR Sec. 483.35]

The regulations address several areas that affect how the facility might be expected to meet that requirement.

1. **Staffing.** A qualified dietician must be available on a full-time, part-time, or consultative basis. The facility is also required to have enough staff to carry out the nutritional program, that is, to prepare and serve the meals in adequate portions and in timely fashion so that the food is not undercooked, overcooked, or served too cold or too hot.

2. **Nutritional adequacy and menu planning.** The dietician must design the menu offerings to meet the nutritional requirements of all the residents, based on the recommended dietary allowances (RDA) of the Food and Nutrition Board of the National Research Council of the National Academy of Sciences. In addition, the facility must provide for the special dietary needs of those with therapeutic diets ordered by their physicians for conditions such as diabetes, heart disease, or high blood pressure and for special consistencies such as soft or blended diets.

3. **Food preparation.** Food must be stored properly and meals must be appealing and prepared to preserve nutritional value. A facility cannot try to keep dietary staff at a bare minimum by using huge meal preparation lead time if it results in food sitting for prolonged periods under heat lamps or on steam tables, resulting in soggy or dried out entrees for the residents.

4. **Substitution.** Nutritionally adequate substitutes are required since residents have the right to refuse the standard menu offering. As mentioned elsewhere, the facility is not required to offer a menu as diverse as a typical restaurant, but it does have to offer palatable

and nutritionally sound alternatives to the main menu. If the resident has therapeutic diet orders, the types of substitutes and preparation preferences may be limited somewhat, but *choice* cannot be eliminated.

5. **Special diets.** *Therapeutic diets* must be prepared to meet the individual's medical needs with as much attention to individual choice as possible. Therapeutic diets are ordered by the physician to reduce or increase certain nutrients in the person's intake. *Mechanically altered diets* may also be ordered to make it easier and safer for residents with chewing or swallowing difficulties to eat.

6. **Frequency of meals.** The facility must provide at least three meals scheduled to be served around the same times prevalent in the community. An evening snack is usually provided because the rules require that not more than 14 hours elapse from the time the last regular meal of the day is served and the time that breakfast is served the next day. The provision by the facility of an evening snack allows the time span to extend to 16 hours.

7. **Sanitation.** Food must be stored, prepared, distributed, and served under sanitary conditions. This rule applies all day, every day, without exception. In addition, foodstuffs must be procured from reputable vendors. Utensils must be cleaned and stored under specified conditions. Waste and refuse must be kept away from food storage, preparation, and handling areas.

Apart from these requirements, the dietary program must be coordinated with the nursing services in the facility to ensure that the resident's health status is being maintained or improved to the greatest extent possible from a nutritional standpoint. This means the facility must achieve several things. First, **clinical nutritional indicators** must be monitored for each resident at risk for nutritional problems. Nutritional risk factors include a history of recent significant weight loss; loss of appetite; difficulties with swallowing or chewing due to stroke, dental problems, surgery, and the like; use of certain medications; depression; and cancer. Further, if an individual is at risk, the facility

must assess for signs of nutritional problems such as weight loss, weakness, muscle wasting, and dry mouth and should consider monitoring food and fluid intake.

Weight loss can become controversial in long-term care facilities. The bottom line is that it is not considered acceptable unless it can reasonably be related to a clinical condition that would make preventing the weight loss impossible. However, even if that is the case, the facility must continue to assess the problem and try to address it.

■
WAGING WAR ON WEIGHT LOSS

According to statistics from the Health Care Financing Administration Center for Information Systems, 3.6 percent of nursing home residents had reportable weight gain or loss in 1995. That figure may not make weight loss appear to be a common problem; however, it presumably reflects only the number of individuals with *significant* or *severe* weight loss, based on the following criteria.

The rules provide guidelines for assessing the severity of weight loss and what to do about it. They suggest that a 5 percent weight loss in one month is significant, greater than that is severe; a 7.5 percent weight loss in three months is significant, greater than that is severe; a 10 percent weight loss in six months is significant, greater than that is severe. The rules also suggest certain values for selected laboratory tests that can be used to evaluate nutritional status, but the rules *do not require* that the lab work be done.

Weight reduction may be a *therapeutic* outcome. In that case, the physician will order the calorie level designed to cause gradual weight loss; you should be made aware of this and agree to it as part of the care plan. However, when *unplanned* weight loss is occurring, the facility should assess the possible causes for it and the facility need not necessarily wait until the weight loss is at a level where it could be considered significant or severe before looking for causes and solutions.

To help you become an active partner with the facility staff in preventing weight loss, malnutrition, and dehydration, here are some of the key warning signs to watch for:

1. Pale, dry-looking skin. The skin may also be very thin, fragile, and inelastic, prone to bruising or injury. (If you note bruising or injuries such as skin tears, discuss them with the nursing supervisors. If you are the decision maker, you should be notified of any incidents that result in injury.)

2. "Tenting" of the skin, called "poor skin turgor." This is tested for by gently pinching the skin on the back of the hand up into a "tent" for a few seconds and releasing. If the skin stays in a tent shape or retracts back flat very slowly, it may indicate dehydration.

3. Dry mouth and dull appearing eyes.

4. Confusion or other changes in alertness.

5. Weakness, unsteadiness in walking, or dizziness when standing up.

6. Appearance of "sunken eyes," visible muscle wasting, clothing appearing to fit more loosely.

7. Muscle twitching, or complaints of muscle pain or cramps.

8. Dull, dry-looking hair and hair loss.

9. Tooth loss, red, swollen gums, or bleeding from the gums.

When unplanned weight loss occurs, especially immediately after the person is admitted to the facility, it may be due to a loss of appetite because of the multitude of changes taking place as a result of the move to the nursing home itself. That situation should be expected to be temporary, and a policy of "watchful waiting" may be called for. Once a degree of stability and familiarity is established, appetite may return and the weight loss reversed. The facility may simply need to monitor body weight and intake of food and fluids for a time to establish that this is the case. Many facilities routinely do this for people who are newly admitted. Ask the facility for its policy on weight monitoring to find out if this is the case.

However, if unplanned weight loss continues and physical signs and symptoms are becoming evident, assessment of causes should occur and the care plan should reflect some action to stop and reverse the trend of weight loss. There are some things consumers should expect the facility to consider as it assesses the possible causes for weight loss, and there are some actions consumers should expect the facility to take in response when those causes are identified.

Problem 1. Weight loss despite a good appetite (eating well at every meal and snacks).

What can be done about it?

1. Dietary assessment: Are enough calories and protein being provided? Enough fluids?

2. Nursing assessment: Nausea, vomiting, diarrhea, or constipation occurring? Medication changes? Check blood glucose (for adult-onset diabetes). Monitor weight weekly.

3. Physician assessment: Lab work, including blood work to determine if anemia, thyroid problems, or protein deficiencies are present. Physical assessment for abnormalities such as malabsorption syndrome (a condition which causes the body to be unable to use nutrients in the food) or cancer.

Problem 2. Poor intake (not taking most or any of the food or fluids being offered).

What can be done about it?

1. Dietary assessment: Do the menu offerings appeal to the person? Are substitutes being offered? Are the menu items culturally appropriate? Special diet ordered (therapeutic or mechanically altered)? If adaptive utensils are required, are they being provided?

2. Nursing assessment: Mood changes or signs of depression? Medication changes? Problems with dentition (bad teeth or gums), chewing, or swallowing? Nausea, vomiting, diarrhea or constipation occurring? Inadequate time to eat, e.g., not being given enough help, if that is necessary, due to short staffing? Meals interrupted by other residents or staff? Ordered supplements not being given? Calorie count (detailed evaluation of food intake) and weekly weights may need to be done.

3. Social services assessment: Problems with adjustment to the facility? Family or other personal/financial issues? Problems with tablemates at meals?

4. Physician assessment: Medication side effects or interactions? Untreated depression? Physical evaluation, lab work, or specialist consultation may be needed. In very serious cases, the use of intravenous (IV) fluids or nutrients or a feeding tube may be considered (see chapter 17).

These lists are not comprehensive—there are a lot of issues that can contribute to unplanned weight loss in the nursing home. The key message here is that something can be done to deal with most of them and there should always be a thorough assessment of what is causing unplanned weight loss and dehydration problems.

7

Protecting Your Rights in the Long-Term Care Setting

In a nation with a strong democratic tradition, you would expect your rights and the exercise of those rights to be protected whether or not you live in a long-term care facility. Because this is not always the case, OBRA provides a very specialized bill of rights that applies to individuals living in long-term-care facilities. This chapter introduces these very important rights. Although it provides a condensed version of OBRA, it is more detailed than the bill of rights most facilities provide.

Typically, individuals who are admitted to long-term care facilities have been through a serious illness, injury, or major surgery. Indeed, fully 68 percent of the people admitted to long-term care facilities come directly from acute care hospitals. Others suffer with a cognitive impairment such as Alzheimer's disease or another form of dementia. They are usually physically weakened or intellectually impaired, or they may be dealing with both problems at the same time. Simply stated, they may be vulnerable to financial exploitation, physical, verbal, emotional, or sexual abuse, neglect, or intimidation. This chapter describes protections for the rights of long-term care residents and how to enforce them.

Admission to a long-term care facility can be frightening and confusing. Intensifying the difficulty of this event are the concerns one may have about his or her own health or that of a loved one being admitted. One may also sense a loss of control, including loss of control over everyday routines such as what and when to eat or what to wear, and perhaps loss of control over finances, role in one's family, and health care decision making.

Federal and state laws have been written to help preserve a resident's right to maintain the highest degree of control possible over these issues while residing in a nursing home.

■

THE RESIDENT'S BILL OF RIGHTS

1. You have the right to exercise your rights as a citizen of the United States and of your state and as a resident of the facility in which you reside. Most facilities will have a written **Resident's Bill of Rights.** It must be provided to you upon admission to the facility, and if the facility does not offer it, *insist* on it. If you visit the facility in advance of being admitted as part of selecting the right nursing home, be sure to request a copy. (See chapter 5, "Choosing a Long-Term Care Facility.")

2. You have the right to be free of any interference, coercion (pressure), discrimination of any kind, threat of reprisal, or retaliation by the facility as the result of your exercise of any of your rights. For example, the facility may not interfere with your right to file a complaint about the facility by denying you access to a telephone or writing materials.

3. You have the right to be informed *in writing* of your rights as a resident in the facility. You must be informed in writing of the rules you are expected to follow while living in the facility. The law requires that you acknowledge receipt of this information in writing. However, obtaining your signature is *not enough*. To be in full compliance with the law, the facility must explain your rights and the rules orally in terms you can understand.

The law specifically requires that the facility overcome barriers to understanding that the resident may have, such as speaking a foreign language or severe vision or hearing impairment. This may include having the bill of rights printed in translations appropriate to the situation, using an interpreter, or having large-print versions of the information available.

It is important not to rush through this information. This information and knowing how to use it can help ensure a satisfying, safe, and cost-effective care experience in the long-term care facility. Simply put, if you do not fully understand your rights and the facility rules, the facility has failed to meet this requirement.

4. You have the right to free choice with respect to selecting a physician, receiving or declining treatment, refusing to participate in any experimental research, and you have the right to participate in making decisions concerning your care.

5. You have the right to privacy and confidentiality. This includes your right to personal privacy in communications,

visitation, and association. It means that all personal and clinical records will be held in strictest confidence to the extent allowed by law. You may refuse to release records to a third party except when the records are necessary for transfer of your care to another facility, by law, or by third-party payment contract (such as your insurance company or Medicare). This right does not require the facility to provide a private room.

Violations of the right to privacy are among the most common infractions that occur in nursing homes. (See chapter 15, "Hear My Voice," for more on this important issue.)

6. You have the right to voice grievances or complaints about the facility and to have the facility respond to them. The facility must act in good faith on your complaints and must ensure that there is no reprisal or discrimination against the anyone who files a complaint or grievance. The facility must act promptly to resolve issues raised in a complaint. (See also "What Happens When You File a Complaint about Suspected Abuse?" in chapter 22, "Freedom from Abuse, Neglect, and Fear," for related information.)

7. You have the right to examine the results of state and federal surveys of the facility. The results of the most recent annual survey report must be readily accessible to residents, their families, or decision makers. Look for a form called "Statement of Deficiencies" (HCFA form 2567) and the statement of isolated deficiencies (if any).

The survey reports tend to be technical in the way they are written. If there are any aspects of the survey report or, perhaps more important, any aspects of the facility's plan of correction (written on the right-hand side of the HCFA form 2567) that you question or do not understand, ask the facility's director of social services, director of nursing, or administrator to explain it.

In addition, the facility must provide information about agencies that act as resident advocates, such as the state survey agency, bureau of quality assurance, long-term care ombudsman's offices, or state office on aging. (Of course, since you have this book, you only need to turn directly to appendixes G, I, and J for this information.) You must be afforded the opportunity to contact these agencies, if you should wish to do so.

8. You have the right to work or *not to work* while living in a long-term care facility. You have the right to refuse to perform any services for the facility or, if you choose to, you may work for the facility when work is included in your care plan, the plan specifies what you will be doing and whether it is on an unpaid volunteer basis or for pay, in which case the rate paid must equal or exceed the prevailing rates for such work, and you must agree to do the work in the care plan.

9. You have the right to privacy in sending and receiving mail. Your mail must not be opened without your consent and must be delivered to you promptly (within 24 hours of the Postal Service delivering it to the facility); your outgoing mail must be delivered to the post office within the same time period.

10. You have the right to visit and be visited by others and to refuse to allow access to certain individuals. While facilities have the right to set reasonable visiting hours, they may not restrict access to residents by immediate family members, unless the resident requests it. The facility may specify where visits take place if other residents or roommates would normally be sleeping at the time of the visits.

The facility may not restrict access to residents by any representative of the Secretary of Health and Human Services, any representative of the state, the resident's physician, the state long-term care ombudsman, or representatives from advocacy agencies for the mentally retarded or mentally ill. Though the rules say a resident may not refuse to see a state surveyor (an official who inspects nursing homes), I have never seen a state surveyor ignore the wishes of a resident who was considered competent to make decisions.

Other parties, such as representatives of agencies which provide health, legal, social, or other services to the resident, can be granted "reasonable access" subject to the facility's policies and the impact of such access on the privacy rights and delivery of care for other residents.

11. You have the right to have privacy in your communications by telephone. This means you not only have access to a phone in the facility, but you also have the right to be able to use it in privacy to the extent that your conversations are not overheard. If the resident does not have a private phone in his or her room, phones in staff offices that are not in use, cordless phones, or other access must be available. A public pay phone in the facility lobby or hallway and the phone at the nurses' station generally are not considered adequate to meet this requirement.

12. You have the right to retain and use personal possessions to the greatest extent possible. As space in the room allows, the facility must allow residents to keep and use personal items such as furniture and clothing, provided they do not infringe on the rights or jeopardize the safety of other residents. Thus a resident may bring in a favorite rocking chair if it can fit safely in the room and does not interfere with the delivery of care, but that old desk-top radio with the frayed power cord—a potential fire hazard—is not allowed.

Also, on the subject of personal possessions, be aware that valuable items are always in danger of being stolen. Most facilities encourage residents to place valuables—jewelry, heirlooms, medals, and the like—in the facility safe rather than keeping them in their room, or better yet, to not have those items brought to the facility at all. This provision prevents the facility from prohibiting residents from keeping personal possessions in their room, but bear in mind that the possibility of loss or theft does exist even in the finest facilities.

13. You have the right to be informed about the facility policies for protecting your personal funds in the facility's possession.

14. You have the right to live with your spouse in the same room if that is agreeable to both. This does not mean that a resident can force the facility to relocate another resident to accommodate a spouse; rather, it calls for the facility to allow a married couple to share a room when such an arrangement can be made and only if both partners agree to do so. In addition, the payer source for each partner may be a factor; for example, if only one spouse or the other requires skilled nursing care under the Medicare program and for that reason qualifies to be in the facility's certified distinct part (a separate Medicare-certified area of the facility), the room-sharing arrangement may not be possible unless the spouse who does not require skilled nursing agrees to pay for the stay in the room.

15. You have the right to self-administer your medications if you are able to do so safely. This means the facility must document an evaluation by the care-planning team (of which the resident or the resident's decision maker is a part) as to the resident's ability to self-administer medications. Many people enter a nursing home with the mistaken notion that "the nurse gives me my medications and that's part of what they get paid for." The nurses are there to administer medications to residents who cannot do this safely on their own. The mission of the nursing home these days is to maintain or return those in its care to their highest level of function and independence, which includes taking medications. Remaining independent in taking medications is one of the key criteria that can help set the stage for going home.

16. You have the right to refuse to transfer from your room in a facility's Medicare-certified distinct part to a noncertified part of the building. This can occur when a resident's condition improves to the point where skilled nursing as defined in the Medicare program is no longer required or the Medicare coverage runs out. This right prevents the facility from simply moving a resident out of a room in the certified distinct part of the building unless the resident consents to the room change, even if the resident no longer qualifies for coverage under the Medicare program. Also, if a resident occupies a bed in a part of the facility approved for the *Medicaid* program, the resident cannot be transferred against his or her will by either the facility or the state to a bed in the Medicare-certified portion of the building in order to have the Medicare program pay for the care. A resident may request such a change voluntarily, however. For the purposes of this right, the term **transfer** can also refer to the movement of a resident from one facility to another. The term **discharge** refers to the movement of a resident from a facility to a noninstitutional setting, generally the resident's

home. If a facility pressures a resident to make such a room change inappropriately, it may constitute a violation of this right. If a resident chooses to exercise this right, eligibility for the Medicare or Medicaid program is not affected.

Generally, a facility may not transfer or discharge a resident unless

a. The facility cannot meet the resident's welfare needs.

b. The resident's condition has improved to the point where the facility's services are no longer needed.

c. The safety or health of individuals in the facility is threatened.

d. The resident has failed to pay for care in the facility and reasonable notice has been given.

e. The facility ceases to operate.

If the facility does intend to transfer someone to another facility or discharge a resident, it is required to do certain things before the discharge or transfer takes place:

a. Notify the resident, family member, or decision maker at least 30 days in advance, or as soon as possible, depending on the reason for the discharge or transfer.

b. Provide in the notification the reason(s) for the action, the date it will occur, the location to which the discharged or transferred person is to go, information about the right to appeal the decision and how to contact the state's long-term care ombudsman's office, (see appendix J), and information about how to reach appropriate protective or advocacy agencies.

c. The facility must prepare and orient the resident to ensure a safe and orderly discharge or transfer. This may include involving residents and their families or decision makers in the planning process to the greatest extent possible, arranging an orientation tour or visit to the receiving facility in the case of a transfer, and providing detailed orientation to caregivers of the facility taking over the resident's care as to the resident's daily patterns, preferences, and needs.

d. The facility must provide written notice of the facility's bed-hold policy to residents, their families, or decision makers if the transfer is for hospitalization or for a therapeutic leave. Remember to look for the duration of the bed hold and how many days may be covered as part of your long-term care coverage in your private insurance or your state Medicaid program. You must understand at what point you would be required to pay for a bed hold.

e. The facility must provide its policy on readmission when the leave or hospitalization exceeds the number of days specified in the state Medicaid program.

17. You have the right to be informed of your eligibility status with respect to Medicaid benefits, the time at which you become eligible for Medicaid, those items and services covered under Medicaid, those things the program does not cover, and what the resident can be charged for and how much the facility charges for those goods and services; the resident also must be informed of any changes to the services provided and the charges for them.

18. You have the right to be informed prior to the time of admission of what services are available in the facility, what they cost, and which services are covered and not covered by the Medicare program or which services are not included in the facility's per diem (daily charge) rate.

19. You have the right to know the names of physicians involved in providing care and how to reach them.

20. You have the right to be informed about the Medicare and Medicaid programs and how to apply for benefits under those programs.

21. You have the right to be fully informed about your plan of care and treatment and to have input into decisions affecting your care. In the event a resident is not mentally competent to make care and treatment decisions, the resi-

dent's designated decision maker or family member must be informed about the plan of care and allowed to participate in care planning. More about this appears in chapter 8, "For the Record: Your Right to See Your Medical Record," and chapter 17, "Advance Directive: Terms of Empowerment."

22. You (or family members or decision makers) have the right to be informed promptly about changes of condition or status, including:

a. Any accident or incident which results in injury to the resident.

b. A significant change in condition including changes in mental, physical, or psychosocial status.

c. The need to significantly change the plan of care or treatment.

d. The decision to transfer or discharge the resident.

e. Plans to change room or roommate.

f. Changes to residents' rights under state or federal law.

23. You have the right to manage your personal finances. The facility cannot require residents to deposit personal funds with the facility. If the resident requests the facility to manage his or her funds, the facility may not refuse, but the facility is not responsible for knowing about funds not on deposit with it. Each resident's funds may be in a separate account or funds may be combined with other funds. If accounts are pooled, interest is prorated per individual on the basis of actual earnings or end-of-quarter balance.

Funds not exceeding $50 ($100 for residents being covered by the Medicare program) must be kept in separate, interest- or non–interest-bearing accounts or a petty cash fund. Resident requests for access to funds of $50 or less ($100 for Medicare residents) must be honored the same day. Requests for greater amounts must be honored within three banking days. Funds exceeding $50 ($100 for residents covered by Medicare) must be deposited in interest-bearing accounts, not the facility's operating accounts, and interest must be credited to the resident's account.

The facility must provide a written record of the account upon the request of the resident or decision maker. The facility must use an accounting system that precludes combining resident fund amounts with facility funds or those of other residents. The facility must report the fund balances to the resident or decision maker at least quarterly. **Note:** The facility must notify Medicaid recipients

a. When the amount in their account reaches less than $200 of the single-person resource limit, and

b. That if the amount in the account combined with the value of the resident's other nonexempt resources exceeds the single-person resource limit, the resident may lose eligibility for Medicaid or Supplemental Security Income (SSI).

In the event of a resident's death, the facility must, within 30 days, convey the resident's funds with a final accounting statement to the individual or probate jurisdiction administering the resident's estate.

The facility must ensure the security of resident funds under its control by a surety bond or other acceptable method. (A surety bond is an insurance policy that protects the resident from suffering a financial loss as the result of the facility's failure to safeguard, manage, or account for the resident's funds.) While the rules do allow some alternative approaches to a surety bond, they do not allow the facility to use self-insurance or to consider deposits placed in an account insured by the FDIC (Federal Deposit Insurance Corporation) as alternatives to meet this requirement.

Finally, under this right, the facility is prohibited from making a charge against resident funds for any item or service that is covered under Medicare or Medicaid, except for any copay amounts or deductibles that may apply. The facility may *not* charge residents for any of the following categories of items and services:

a. Nursing services.

b. Dietary services.

c. Activities (recreation therapy) services.

d. Room or bed maintenance services.

e. Routine personal hygiene items, over-the-counter drugs, and laundry services.

f. Medically related social services.

There are some categories of items and services you may be charged for, even if you are in the Medicare or Medicaid program. If the facility provides a good or service for which there will be a charge, you or your decision maker must be informed of that and what the charge will be. These services include:

a. Telephone in your room.

b. Television or radio for personal use.

c. Personal comfort items, candy, smoking materials, and so on.

d. Cosmetic or grooming items not paid for by Medicare or Medicaid.

e. Personal clothing or reading materials.

f. Gifts purchased on behalf of a resident.

g. Flowers and plants.

h. Social events or entertainment not included in the facility's activity program.

i. Private-duty nurses or aides.

j. Private rooms except when medically necessary for isolation.

k. Specially prepared foods not otherwise offered by the facility, but the facility may not charge a resident for a special diet which is medically necessary and ordered by the resident's physician.

24. You have the right to equal access to quality care. Facilities must treat all residents alike where decisions about transfers and discharge are concerned. Facilities must not distinguish between residents based on their source of payment when providing services that are required by law. All nursing services, specialized rehabilitative services, dietary services, social services, pharmaceutical services, and activities that are mandated by law must be provided to residents based on the assessment of their needs and their care plan *irrespective of the resident's payer source.*

25. You have the right to coverage without additional conditions. Note the following:

a. A facility may not request or require residents or potential residents to waive their rights to coverage under the Medicare or Medicaid program as a condition for admission. Further, a facility may not require residents or potential residents to give oral or written assurance that they will not apply for Medicare or Medicaid benefits.

b. A facility may not require a third-party guarantee of payment (this refers to payment by a person such as a relative, not to payment by a third-party payer such as an insurance company) as a condition of admission or of continued stay in the facility. The resident's authorized family member or decision maker may, however, be allowed to sign a contract to pay for the facility's services from the resident's financial resources.

c. For individuals eligible for Medicaid-covered services, a facility may not solicit, charge, or accept any gift, money or consideration, or donation for any amount in excess of the payment made by Medicaid for the facility's services as a condition for admission. This not to say the facility cannot accept charitable contributions. It can accept donations as long as they are not made by an individual with a relationship to a Medicaid-eligible resident or potential resident and

the contribution is not a condition of admission or continued stay in the facility.

26. You have the right to be free of any physical or chemical restraint imposed for the purpose of discipline or convenience; this does not include restraint required to *treat your symptoms.* The use of physical restraints and psychoactive drugs (chemical restraints) are two major reasons nursing home reform was initiated. Physical restraints and the issues they raise are covered in chapter 21, "Don't Tie Me Down! The Right to Be Free from the Use of Physical Restraints." Chapter 20, "Powerful Stuff: Rules That Protect You from Misuse of Psychoactive Medications," covers chemical restraints in detail. An important feature in those chapters is the discussion of criteria for assessment to determine if the use of restraints or drugs is necessary and a discussion of possible alternatives to the use of each.

27. You have the right to be free from physical, verbal, sexual, and mental abuse, corporal punishment, and involuntary seclusion. See chapter 22, "Freedom from Abuse, Neglect, and Fear," for a detailed discussion of the rules designed to protect you from abuse.

28. You have the right to be cared for in a manner that promotes and maintains your quality of life. The facility must provide or ensure the following:

a. Dignity and individuality.

b. Self-determination and participation in activities or associations of your choosing.

c. Ability to meet your own needs or have individual needs accommodated by the facility.

d. An activities program that meets your interests and needs.

e. Medically related social services to help you attain or maintain the highest possible level of physical, mental, and psychosocial well-being.

Chapters 13, 14, and 15 deal with these protections in more detail.

29. You have the right to live in a safe, clean, homelike environment (see chapter 6).

Some of the following chapters expand on key areas that you need to know about. If you have questions or problems with the way a facility manages your care or that of a loved one and you believe these rights are being violated, discuss it with the administration of the facility at once. Make it clear to the facility that if a necessary action is not taken, you will seek the assistance of regulatory agencies or the state ombudsman's office.

8

For the Record

You have the right to see and obtain a copy of your medical records. You or your legal representative has the right to have access to all of your medical and financial records that the facility possesses upon your oral or written request. The facility must produce the records within 24 hours of your request, not including weekends or holidays. The facility cannot require your request be in writing if you simply want to read your medical record—an oral request has to be enough. Most facilities will require that a request for copies of your record be in writing, though, and this is permissible.

Your medical record, also referred to as your "chart," is generally considered to include the portion of the medical record that is kept in a binder of one sort or another on the nursing unit at the nurse's station. If you, or your decision maker, family member, or designated legal representative, want to have access to any portion of your medical record that may have been removed from the chart as part of a "chart-thinning" process, be sure to specify that you wish to see the *complete* record, including any purged or old records.

■
What Is in the Chart?

The typical chart will contain the following types of records:

1. A cover sheet with your personal (called demographic) information.

2. A section for the originals of signed physicians' orders.

3. The signed originals of physicians' progress notes.

4. Original nurses' notes.

5. Consultant notes (if any), including mental health or consultant pharmacist notes.

6. Original social services notes.

7. A copy of the history and physical examination (often referred to as the H&P) performed around the time of admission to the facility.

8. A copy of the hospital discharge summary and other hospital records that may have been sent from the hospital providing care just prior to admission to the long-term care facility, if that is where the resident was admitted from. If the person was in the care of another facility such as a nursing home or home health agency, there should be some transfer records from that entity.

9. Originals of the most recent medication administration records (called the MARs). These sheets are usually kept on the medication cart until they are filled out for the period they are designed to cover, usually a month; then they are kept in the chart for a month or two, when they are removed from the chart binder and placed in a file as part of the "old" record. The flow of this process can vary considerably from facility to facility.

10. Original therapy notes, such as physical, occupational, speech, and respiratory therapy, if applicable to the care being given.

11. A section with the original slips with lab results.

12. A section for X-ray reports.

13. A section with the individualized care plan.

14. Dietary services assessment notes.

15. The detailed standardized assessment tool mandated in OBRA called the MDS, or Minimum Data Set. (See chapter 9, "The Minimum Data Set: Getting to Know You.")

16. A portion of the Minimum Data Set called the Resident Assessment Protocol (RAP), which helps guide the assessment process to greater levels of detail based on items in the MDS, where responses based on the assessment "trigger" the need for more detailed assessment. Also present is a document called the "trigger legend," indicating which items in the MDS were triggers and potential triggers for detailed assessment.

Other documents that may show up in the chart include:

1. Specialized forms used for reporting the facility's monitoring of the resident for the side effects of psychoactive drugs. (See chapter 20, "Powerful Stuff: Rules That Protect You from Misuse of Psychoactive Medications," for more detail on this.)

2. Legal documents dealing with advance directives, guardianship papers, and a copy of a durable power of attorney for health care, if you have one.

3. Consent forms for treatments, the use of physical restraints, and often for the use of psychoactive medications.

4. The admission contract and other forms signed at the time of admission.

5. Flow sheets or monitoring records such as IV fluid records, dietary intake records, weight tracking records, enteral feeding records (if tube feeding is taking place), intake and output (I&O) records, turning and repositioning records, physical restraint release records (used to document that physical restraints have been checked and released, and the restrained person has been given the opportunity to walk and use the toilet), and behavioral monitoring records. There may also be records of the treatment of specific conditions such as skin breakdown. A number of the day-to-day flow sheets just listed are not filled out by licensed nursing staff. They are generally filled out by the certified nursing staff or other staff. They are often very revealing about how well things are going for the resident and how consistently basic elements of the care plan are being carried out. Requesting to see these types of records is a worthwhile thing to do when evaluating the plan of care. Some of them can be a little daunting, so do not be afraid to ask the facility staff to help you interpret them.

6. For individuals who have been in the facility for approximately 90 days, there will be a variation of the Minimum Data Set called the Quarterly Review, which is a format for doing a standardized reassessment of some key areas of resident condition. Of course, as the name implies, this assessment is to be done quarterly,

and changes noted as a result of the Quarterly Review that would make revision of the care plan necessary should, in fact, result in changes to the care plan. The resident or the decision maker must have the opportunity to contribute to the Quarterly Review and sign off on it.

It is a good idea to go over the chart with a member of the facility staff who can answer your questions about the record itself, help find information for you (this is really important, since the chart can tend to be a very thick set of documents), and help you understand the technical aspects of your care. Since your record is confidential, you have the right to review it in a place that affords some privacy. You may need to be flexible in terms of scheduling a time to review the chart if you wish to have nursing or therapy staff present. Their time is very tightly scheduled, but do not let them put you off without a good reason. After all, your care or that of your loved one is every bit as important as anyone else's.

If you wish to purchase a copy of the record, or some portion of it, you cannot be denied but you can be charged. The law states that you may not be charged more than the "community standard" cost for a photocopy of your record. Exactly what that means may be dictated by law in your state, but if the law does not specify an amount, the amount may be determined by the cost per page charged by the local post office, public library, or commercial copy center.

You may also be charged for clerical time to actually do the copying, but you may not be charged for locating or "pulling" the record or for typing time. The facility is required to produce the copy of the record in no more than two working days.

KNOW AS YOU GO: HOW TO USE YOUR MEDICAL RECORD TO STAY INFORMED

The ability to choose the path your care will follow and to participate in a meaningful way in the decision-making process depends on *understanding* clinical information about your condition or that of your loved one rather than merely having access to it. This is the area where the long-term care regulations take a long stride beyond most consumer protection laws. The facility must demonstrate not only that it makes the effort to keep residents fully informed about their health status, but that it ensures that residents or their decision makers understand the information.

The facility must document its efforts to inform you of your medical condition, treatment, care plan, and so on, in language or by a means that you or a decision maker understands. In other words, simply giving a resident or family member a preprinted handout describing a condition, treatment, or procedure is not enough—a staff member must explain it as well. To make sure it is clear, the use of technical terms must be minimized to the extent possible and terms that may not be understood must be explained.

Of course, the resident or decision maker has the duty to ask questions if the information being given is not clear. Never be afraid to ask questions and do not settle for anything less than a clear answer. The facility staff may refer some medical issues to the attending physician, and that is fine. The physician plays a lead role in your care and is often the best source for information.

YOU MUST BE NOTIFIED OF CHANGES

The facility is required to notify the resident and/or family member or decision maker and the attending physician about significant changes that affect your condition, care, or living arrangements. A resident who is his or her own decision maker, may specify that family members be notified or not notified, but that needs to be expressed *in writing* to avoid any confusion about who should be told what. If a resident wishes to withhold information about a condition from any specific individuals, the facility must be informed so that those directions can be noted in the chart. Specifically, the facility must provide notification of any of the following changes:

1. An accident or other incident resulting in injury.

2. A significant change in mental or physical condition.

3. The need to make a significant change to the care plan or treatment.

4. The decision to discharge or transfer a resident and the reasons for the decision.

5. Any change of room or roommate.

6. Any change of resident's rights under state or federal law.

A great way to stay informed about changes is to establish a strong informal relationship with facility staff. Getting to know staff members on a personal level can facilitate ongoing communication and foster trust and confidence. This can be difficult if you are a decision maker living far from the facility and visit the facility only periodically, but it can be of greatest value under those circumstances as well.

9

The Minimum Data Set

GETTING TO KNOW YOU
(AND WHY THAT IS IMPORTANT)

Prior to the introduction of the Minimum Data Set (MDS) as a part of the OBRA reforms, nursing homes developed their own admission physical assessment forms and procedures to follow. This resulted in a hodgepodge of ways of gathering baseline data on a new resident, with most methods focusing on physical assessment only, seeking to record baseline vital signs and often not much more. The personal habits, interests, cultural background, and daily living patterns of the new resident were often overlooked. Since the psychological, social, and emotional state of the *person* being cared for often went unnoticed and undocumented, those aspects of care for that person tended to be overlooked from then on.

The lack of consistency in assessment made it difficult for family members, decision makers, physicians, and state surveyors (facility inspectors) to know for sure how the person was doing at the time of admission as a basis for comparison to how the resident was progressing as a result of the facility's care.

Some facilities had excellent documentation of *physical* indicators—vital signs, lung sounds, wound dimensions, and so on—but nothing on the person's mental state, that is, cognitive (intellectual) state or emotional well-being. Some facilities documented an excellent history of the present episode of illness, did a poor job of assessing the person's other medical history, and did nothing at all in terms of assessing the person's lifestyle preferences, interests, and abilities prior to illness. The absence of this information meant that facilities tended to focus their energy on the most recent diagnosis and on the technical aspects of the care they would provide. The *person* in their care was in danger of being overlooked. The human needs tended to be underestimated if they were considered at all.

Beyond the initial assessment, there often was no consistent use of the information that was gathered. The care plan that should be based on the integration of all information pertinent to the person's problems and needs all too often was sketchy, disjointed, and incomplete. Goals for the resident's care, if stated at all, were often irrelevant or unrealistic. Ongoing assessment of the resident's condition and needs tended to be irregular or disorganized, or it did not happen at all.

These issues played a role in the creation of a uniform assessment system for use by long-term care facilities called the **Resident Assessment Instrument (RAI).** The RAI was introduced along with the rest of OBRA in 1987. The use of the RAI or a federally approved equivalent is mandatory. States are free to make additions or improvements to the instrument in Section S of the MDS, to make them "state-specific" if they wish, but those changes require federal approval.

The RAI includes four key elements:

1. The **Minimum Data Set (MDS)** is the standard form that is intended to guide the assessment process down a consistent path and to provide for consistent documentation of the results. As the name suggests, the Minimum Data Set is just that—it is considered to be the *minimum* data the facility is expected to gather as a part of the initial assessment. The expectation on the part of the creators of OBRA is that the facility will exceed the parameters of the MDS in any areas of the resident's assessment that may require it. That is a good thing because the most recent version of the MDS, called MDS 2.0 version (01/30/98) as good as it is, would still allow some physical assessment data to be overlooked if the facility stuck to the letter of the form.

2. The **trigger legend** is the tool designed to help the facility identify which responses on the MDS may or definitely will require further in-depth assessment work using the next tool, called the Resident Assessment Protocols.

3. The **Resident Assessment Protocol (RAP)** is a detailed, step-by-step guideline for further assessment of those items that the trigger legend indicates require it based on what was found during the completion of the Minimum Data Set. The RAP is perhaps the best part of the entire RAI because it provides excellent guidance on how to explore clinically complex care issues in an organized way. The RAP also suggests areas for further assessment that may not have been considered without its use. In this way, RAP can materially improve the care planning that is done and, as a result, improve the care that is actually given. The system uses what is called a RAP Summary Sheet, which identifies the areas of the assessment that triggered further assessment, where that further assessment is documented in the record, the date of the assessment, and whether it resulted in any actions as part of the resident's care plan. Another feature of the RAP is a handy tool for assessing the resident's functional status (ability to perform) basic living skills called **activities of daily living (ADL).** This is one of the most important areas of assessment, requiring an accurate baseline since it gives the some of the most significant information about the resident's progress toward independence.

4. The **Quarterly Review** is basically a condensed version of the MDS that requires the reassessment of some key resident condition indicators. It is the minimum requirement of the RAI, which addresses the need for some form of consistent, periodic review of the case by mandating that the resident be reassessed every three months. Of course, the Quarterly Review is the *least frequent* assessment the facility is expected to do. If a "significant change of condition" occurs, that must result in an entirely new assessment using the full MDS.

I will not go into greater detail about the mechanics of the completion of the MDS and the assessment process. A sample page of the MDS is reproduced here (see p. 82) to help you identify the form in the medical record. The instructions to the facility on how to use these items fill a book in themselves, but this should help you get a clearer view of the assessment and the care planning process.

The Balanced Budget Act of 1997 brought entirely new and major implications to the use of the MDS. Beginning in July 1998, payment for skilled nursing services under the Medicare program is made using a **prospective payment system (PPS).** The PPS is called a "case-mix adjusted pricing system" because the nursing home is supposed to be paid based on the actual resources used to provide care for each resident. This part of the system is based on the resource utilization groups (RUGs) that were developed dur-

MINIMUM DATA SET (MDS) — *VERSION 2.0*
FOR NURSING HOME RESIDENT ASSESSMENT AND CARE SCREENING
FULL ASSESSMENT FORM
(Status in last 7 days, unless other time frame indicated)

SECTION A. IDENTIFICATION AND BACKGROUND INFORMATION

1. RESIDENT NAME

a. (First)   b. (Middle Initial)   c. (Last)   d. (Jr/Sr)

2. ROOM NUMBER

3. ASSESS-MENT REFERENCE DATE
a. Last day of MDS observation period

Month — Day — Year

b. Original (0) or corrected copy of form (enter number of correction)

4a. DATE OF REENTRY
Date of reentry from most recent temporary discharge to a hospital in last 90 days (or since last assessment or admission if less than 90 days)

Month — Day — Year

5. MARITAL STATUS
1. Never married   3. Widowed   5. Divorced
2. Married   4. Separated

6. MEDICAL RECORD NO.

7. CURRENT PAYMENT SOURCES FOR N.H. STAY
(Billing Office to indicate; *check all that apply in last 30 days*)

Medicaid per diem	a.	VA per diem	f.
Medicare per diem	b.	Self or family pays for full per diem	g.
Medicare ancillary part A	c.	Medicaid resident liability or Medicare co-payment	h.
Medicare ancillary part B	d.	Private insurance per diem (including co-payment)	i.
CHAMPUS per diem	e.	Other per diem	j.

8. REASONS FOR ASSESS-MENT
[Note—If this is a discharge or reentry assessment, only a limited subset of MDS items need be completed]

a. Primary reason for assessment
1. Admission assessment (required by day 14)
2. Annual assessment
3. Significant change in status assessment
4. Significant correction of prior full assessment
5. Quarterly review assessment
6. Discharged—return not anticipated
7. Discharged—return anticipated
8. Discharged prior to completing initial assessment
9. Reentry
10. Significant correction of prior quarterly assessment
0. NONE OF ABOVE

b. *Codes for assessments required for Medicare PPS or the State*
1. Medicare 5 day assessment
2. Medicare 30 day assessment
3. Medicare 60 day assessment
4. Medicare 90 day assessment
5. Medicare readmission/return assessment
6. Other state required assessment
7. Medicare 14 day assessment
8. Other Medicare required assessment

9. RESPONSI-BILITY/ LEGAL GUARDIAN
(*Check all that apply*)

Legal guardian	a.	Durable power attorney/financial	d.
Other legal oversight	b.	Family member responsible	e.
Durable power of attorney/health care	c.	Patient responsible for self	f.
		NONE OF ABOVE	g.

10. ADVANCED DIRECTIVES
(*For those items with supporting **documentation** in the medical record, check all that apply*)

Living will	a.	Feeding restrictions	f.
Do not resuscitate	b.	Medication restrictions	g.
Do not hospitalize	c.	Other treatment restrictions	h.
Organ donation	d.	NONE OF ABOVE	i.
Autopsy request	e.		

SECTION B. COGNITIVE PATTERNS

1. COMATOSE
(*Persistent vegetative state/no discernible consciousness*)
0. No   1. Yes   **(If yes, skip to Section G)**

2. MEMORY
(*Recall of what was learned or known*)
a. Short-term memory OK—seems/appears to recall after 5 minutes
0. Memory OK   1. Memory problem
b. Long-term memory OK—seems/appears to recall long past
0. Memory OK   1. Memory problem

3. MEMORY/ RECALL ABILITY
(*Check all that resident was **normally able to recall during last 7 days***)

Current season	a.	That he/she is in a nursing home	d.
Location of own room	b.		
Staff names/faces	c.	NONE OF ABOVE are recalled	e.

4. COGNITIVE SKILLS FOR DAILY DECISION-MAKING
(*Made decisions regarding tasks of daily life*)
0. INDEPENDENT—decisions consistent/reasonable
1. MODIFIED INDEPENDENCE—some difficulty in new situations only
2. MODERATELY IMPAIRED—decisions poor; cues/supervision required
3. SEVERELY IMPAIRED—never/rarely made decisions

5. INDICATORS OF DELIRIUM— PERIODIC DISOR-DERED THINKING/ AWARENESS
(*Code for behavior in the last 7 days.*) [*Note: Accurate assessment requires conversations with staff and family who have direct knowledge of resident's behavior over this time*].
0. Behavior not present
1. Behavior present, not of recent onset
2. Behavior present, over last 7 days appears different from resident's usual functioning (e.g., new onset or worsening)

a. EASILY DISTRACTED—(e.g., difficulty paying attention; gets sidetracked)
b. PERIODS OF ALTERED PERCEPTION OR AWARENESS OF SURROUNDINGS—(e.g., moves lips or talks to someone not present; believes he/she is somewhere else; confuses night and day)
c. EPISODES OF DISORGANIZED SPEECH—(e.g., speech is incoherent, nonsensical, irrelevant, or rambling from subject to subject; loses train of thought)
d. PERIODS OF RESTLESSNESS—(e.g., fidgeting or picking at skin, clothing, napkins, etc; frequent position changes; repetitive physical movements or calling out)
e. PERIODS OF LETHARGY—(e.g., sluggishness; staring into space; difficult to arouse; little body movement)
f. MENTAL FUNCTION VARIES OVER THE COURSE OF THE DAY—(e.g., sometimes better, sometimes worse; behaviors sometimes present, sometimes not)

6. CHANGE IN COGNITIVE STATUS
Resident's cognitive status, skills, or abilities have changed as compared to status of **90 days ago** (or since last assessment if less than 90 days)
0. No change   1. Improved   2. Deteriorated

SECTION C. COMMUNICATION/HEARING PATTERNS

1. HEARING
(*With hearing appliance, if used*)
0. HEARS ADEQUATELY—normal talk, TV, phone
1. MINIMAL DIFFICULTY when not in quiet setting
2. HEARS IN SPECIAL SITUATIONS ONLY—speaker has to adjust tonal quality and speak distinctly
3. HIGHLY IMPAIRED/absence of useful hearing

2. COMMUNI-CATION DEVICES/ TECH-NIQUES
(*Check all that apply* during last 7 days)

Hearing aid, present and used	a.
Hearing aid, present and not used regularly	b.
Other receptive comm. techniques used (e.g., lip reading)	c.
NONE OF ABOVE	d.

3. MODES OF EXPRESSION
(*Check all used* by resident to make needs known)

Speech	a.	Signs/gestures/sounds	d.
Writing messages to express or clarify needs	b.	Communication board	e.
American sign language or Braille	c.	Other	f.
		NONE OF ABOVE	g.

4. MAKING SELF UNDER-STOOD
(*Expressing information content—however able*)
0. UNDERSTOOD
1. USUALLY UNDERSTOOD—difficulty finding words or finishing thoughts
2. SOMETIMES UNDERSTOOD—ability is limited to making concrete requests
3. RARELY/NEVER UNDERSTOOD

5. SPEECH CLARITY
(*Code for speech in the last 7 days*)
0. CLEAR SPEECH—distinct, intelligible words
1. UNCLEAR SPEECH—slurred, mumbled words
2. NO SPEECH—absence of spoken words

6. ABILITY TO UNDER-STAND OTHERS
(*Understanding verbal information content—however able*)
0. UNDERSTANDS
1. USUALLY UNDERSTANDS—may miss some part/intent of message
2. SOMETIMES UNDERSTANDS—responds adequately to simple, direct communication
3. RARELY/NEVER UNDERSTANDS

7. CHANGE IN COMMUNI-CATION/ HEARING
Resident's ability to express, understand, or hear information has changed as compared to status of **90 days ago** (or since last assessment if less than 90 days)
0. No change   1. Improved   2. Deteriorated

☐ = When box blank, must enter number or letter   [a.] = When letter in box, check if condition applies

MDS 2.0 01/30/98

ing the Nursing Home Case-Mix and Quality Demonstration run in six states over several years.

The entire system revolves around the data gathered using the MDS to determine the rate of payment the nursing home will receive. MDS data are plugged into a complex formula that sets the rate of reimbursement for care based on how the care being provided fits into 44 resource utilization groups, a case-mix index (CMI), and the location of the facility (urban vs. rural for factoring in labor cost).

The impact of this pricing system on consumers remains to be seen. Some predict that it will allow facilities to do a better job by paying for all the services they actually provide; others predict the system will run some facilities out of business altogether or result in cutting corners and reduced staffing. It may be that the impact will depend on how well the management of the facility understands the system and adapts to it and how thoroughly the facility's staff complete the MDS.

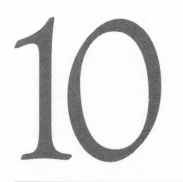

Quality of Care

DEFINING STANDARDS OF CARE

Recognized clinical standards of care or medical practice guidelines that apply to specific types of care or conditions are mandated by some states. OBRA regulations instead establish a definition for professional standards of quality which the survey agency can use to fashion its own interpretation for quality of care and to decide whether a practice is acceptable. Professional standards are defined as

> *Services that are provided according to acceptable standards of clinical practice.*
>
> *[42 CFR Sec.483.20(d)(3)(i)*

These standards of clinical practice may come from professional journals, accreditation standards, clinical practice guidelines published by the Agency for Health Care Policy and Research (AHCPR), standards published by professional associations, rules promulgated by regulatory agencies and licensing authorities, current manuals, and textbooks in the various clinical areas of practice. Standards for each area of clinical specialty that comes into play in long-term care can fill volumes. This fact underscores the importance of the second part of this requirement: What defines a qualified health care practitioner?

Fortunately, this part of the equation is a little clearer, at least from a definition standpoint. A **qualified practitioner** is appropriately licensed or certified by the state to practice his or her specialty in that state, be it medicine, nursing, physical therapy, occupational therapy, speech therapy, respiratory therapy, social work, recreation therapy, dietary or nutrition therapy, pharmacy, psychology, psychiatry, or bedside care as a nursing assistant. Each state requires licensing for nursing home administrators as well.

The facility is responsible for having on hand copies of the licenses of professionals with which it contracts for services and for professional employee staff, including the medical director. Physicians who see patients in the long-term care facility generally do not supply copies of their licenses to those facilities, though the facility could request them. If there are any questions about licensing, the state medical examining board, the local hospital, or your HMO (if you are in one) can help by providing information. Of course, the first person to ask about education, residency, licensing, and board certification of a physician would be the physician. Most physicians are happy to discuss their backgrounds and credentials with their patients or prospective patients.

Most quality-of-care issues for consumers do not arise out of concerns with a clinician's license or whether some clinical protocol has been followed to the letter. The real concerns are more often triggered by attitudes or outcomes. The caregivers who tend to be able to satisfy people's expectations best are often those who take the time to listen to what those in their care have to say. That is true for physicians, therapists, nurses, and nursing assistants. Practitioners should not be judged unfairly by peers and consumers simply because of the difficulty of the workload they had to carry.

Most often, quality-of-care concerns center around the *kind* of care provided or not provided by the physician or the facility. Numbers of staff in the building on each shift are just as likely to be a factor in the quality of care as the training level of each. The quality of services such as dietary and social services also can become the cause of quality problems in a long-term care facility. When dissatisfaction arises, it is best to discuss your concerns with the facility as soon as possible. If there is a medical concern, a conference with the physician may be in order. If there is still a concern about a medical care or treatment issue, you have the right to seek a second opinion, either locally or, if the opinion bears on the need for surgery, call the Second Surgical Opinion Program (see appendix H).

For serious quality-of-care issues that do not receive quick action when presented to the facility, contact the long-term care ombudsman's office in your state (see appendix J), the state survey agency (appendix I), or, for issues involving your doctor, the Medicare professional review organization (PRO), also called quality improvement organization (QIO), in your state (see appendix F).

11

Is There a Doctor in the House?

Who Chooses Your Doctor and What Rules Apply to Physician Services?

When people hear the term "quality of care," they frequently think first about their doctor. Choosing a physician has traditionally been a personal matter, and it has been taken for granted that the patient selects the physician. Unfortunately, these assumptions no longer hold; you should be aware of circumstances that may affect your choice of physician when you enter a long-term care facility.

■ Rights of the Patient

If a person enters a nursing home in his or her hometown, and the person's doctor has a family practice in the community, with numerous mature clients, it is likely that the physician has admitting privileges at most local facilities. In that case, it is likely that the person's regular physician will be able to provide care in the long-term care facility. That is the best situation to be in since the physician is likely to be familiar with the patient's medical history.

There are circumstances, however, when you may not be able to be cared for by the physician you consider to be your regular doctor or you may not have a "regular" doctor or family physician. For example, your doctor may not have admitting privileges at the facility you have been admitted to, or, because of the nature of your care needs, it may be necessary for care to be obtained at a facility outside your home community. This may result in your care being provided outside the normal practice area your doctor serves. If you are in an HMO, the rules of the health plan may delimit the physicians and facilities available for your long-term care needs.

Under such circumstances, the facility will need to assist you in selecting a physician. The facility's social services staff can assist you with this. However, the facility must ensure that you have a physician to give orders for your care *before* your arrival in the facility, leaving little opportunity for you to have meaningful input into the selection process. Indeed, it is not uncommon for the facility to simply select a physician for you.

This does not mean that you have lost the right to choose. If you wish to consider a different physician, the facility must assist you. It must provide you with information about other physicians available to you who are accepting new patients. It also is required to facilitate the process of changing doctors by communicating your wishes to your present doctor and arranging for orders necessary for the transfer of your care.

Planning this aspect of care is a good idea, to the extent that is possible. If you have a regular doctor, find out whether he or she will be able to continue to care for you in the facility you will be admitted to. If, for any reason, the physician will not be able to do so, ask for a recommendation or referral to a physician who can care for you in the facility. This should help give you greater assurance of control of your care and confidence in your choice of physician.

The facility is required to give you information about your physician. This is particularly important if the facility arranged an attending physician for you. You must be informed of the doctor's name and specialty and how to contact the doctor responsible for your care. You have the right to contact the doctor's office *directly* about your care, with *no interference* from the facility. In most instances, it is best to let the facility's nursing or social services staff make contact with the doctor's office in your behalf. This will prevent the doctor's office from getting more than one call on the same subject, avoid confusion, and, in most cases, allow your questions or concerns to be addressed more quickly.

On occasion, the facility may request that a resident change physicians. This request may arise for several reasons: the facility may be preparing to terminate the physician's admitting privileges, the doctor may be failing to comply with the federal or state quality-of-care requirements (more on this later in this chapter), or the physician may be unable to continue to provide care. Under these circumstances, the facility has the responsibility to require that a different doctor assume providing care. The facility must inform residents of this in advance (to the extent possible) and then must assist residents affected by it to select a different doctor.

■

RULES FOR THE DOCTOR

Physician involvement in your care in the long-term care setting must begin before you can be admitted to a facility. A doctor's order is required before anyone can be admitted

to a nursing home, and your care must be under the supervision of a physician on a continuous basis during your stay. Any time the physician designated as your primary care doctor is not available, another physician must be available to direct your care. If possible, it is wise to discuss this in advance with the facility staff or your doctor, so you know the physician's backup should this situation arise. In some cases, the facility's medical director may be called upon to temporarily fill in, and it is a good idea to find out who the medical director is in any case.

OBRA recognizes the key role the physician plays in making the resident's care safe and effective. Consequently, there are some specific rules the physician must follow when caring for a person in the long-term care setting. As an informed consumer or decision maker, you can be the best patient advocate if you feel the physician is not meeting the care needs or is violating the long-term care requirements. The physician must do the following:

1. Evaluate the resident at least every 30 days for the first 90 days after the date of admission and every 60 days thereafter. The physician must actually *see you* during these evaluations. Visits can take place in the doctor's office, if need be, but generally these visits occur when the doctor makes rounds in the facility. In a skilled nursing facility, the doctor may delegate every other visit to a nurse practitioner, clinical nurse specialist, or physician's assistant, if state law allows it. The doctor has a 10-day grace period after the due date for the evaluation in which to complete it, and the doctor does not have the ability to change this requirement. More important than the time requirements for such evaluations are the requirements for what happens during the visit.

2. Review the plan of care, treatments, and medications.

3. Create, sign, and date a progress note that reflects an understanding of the resident's needs and condition; this forms the basis for a decision about whether the plan of care is adequate or appropriate. The progress note should address areas of difficulty in the resident's care or condition as well as areas of improvement. While the doctor is not required to evaluate the entire care plan at each visit, if expected progress has not

taken place, there should be some indication that the physician has reviewed aspects of the care plan that are not working. The simple notation "no new orders" is not adequate.

4. Sign and date all orders generated as a result of the evaluation.

As issues or concerns arise about aspects of your care, or if you simply have questions concerning your care (or your loved one's care), it is a good idea to write them down so they can be discussed when the physician is in the facility on rounds. Of course, urgent questions need not wait: the facility's nursing staff may contact the doctor any time, so do not hesitate to ask them to do so. Never let the staff put things off—your care does not and should not have to wait until the doctor is in on rounds.

When an evaluation performed by a doctor-delegated nurse practitioner, clinical nurse specialist, or physician's assistant finds that a resident's condition warrants a personal evaluation by the physician, that evaluation must happen in timely fashion. Generally, such nonphysician practitioners are known as **physician extenders.** Under OBRA, if they are allowed by state law, they may perform the physi-

cal assessment, review the plan of care, write or dictate a progress note, and sign orders. In some jurisdictions, the physician may need to countersign orders written by physician extenders to demonstrate their supervision of care.

In addition to ensuring that you have a physician to direct your care on a routine basis, the facility is responsible for making sure that you have access to a physician for any emergency care you may require when your attending doctor is not available. Your designation of an alternative doctor ensures that a physician of your choosing is going to care for you. The facility can meet this requirement by arranging transportation for you to the local hospital emergency room when the care you require cannot be provided in the facility.

There are some areas of care that have been given special emphasis in OBRA, and both the facility and the physician have very important roles to play in the compliance with these rules. These areas include the use of physical restraints, psychoactive (sometimes called mood-altering) drugs, unnecessary drugs, and several specific issues that affect both quality of care and quality of life. The key issues in these areas are dealt with in later chapters.

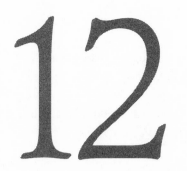

Nurse Aide Training

WHAT CONSUMERS SHOULD
EXPECT THEIR CAREGIVERS
TO KNOW

Some of the finest, most patient, most gracious, and hardest working people I have ever had the pleasure of knowing work in long-term care. As caregivers—nurse aides, certified nursing assistants, nursing assistants, orderlies, nurse aide–registered, competency-evaluated nursing assistants, resident care aides—they have the greatest degree of personal contact with the residents in the facility. No matter the title, they are the people who carry the greatest load of direct care and can have the greatest impact on quality of care and quality of life.

They bathe, dress, turn, and reposition residents who are dependent on others. They brush the teeth or dentures, apply makeup, trim fingernails, do backrubs, and gently flex the joints that some residents cannot flex on their own. They clean up spills, make beds, pick up laundry, clean commodes, and help keep the residents' rooms clean and safe. They are the frontline protection for residents' rights, privacy, and dignity. They listen to complaints, solve problems, offer encouragement and support, and abide working conditions that can be extraordinarily difficult. They are sometimes criticized unfairly, and the depth and difficulty of their work is often poorly understood. Their outlook, attitude, understanding, skill, humor, and patience collectively help to determine the quality of life for those in their care. Because they have more direct contact with each resident than any other discipline in the facility, they can have more influence over the quality of care and quality of life that the resident experiences than anything or anyone else in the building.

The work that they do can be as tedious as it is physically difficult. It can be very hectic, with too many people to care for and too little time and too few hands to help do it. The people in their care can be angry, demanding, insulting, frightening, exasperating, combative, and even dangerous. All these things combined can make the job very stressful, emotionally draining, and physically taxing. On top of it all, these caregivers generally are among the lowest paid staff in the facility.

There is a misbegotten notion in some management circles that anyone can be a nursing assistant in long-term care. This is true to the same extent that anyone can be the president of the United States. The truth is, to do the job in long-term care, it takes a very special person, equipped with a wealth of knowledge and carefully honed skills to do the job right. This is a person with the smiling face whom residents look forward to seeing each day, or whose approaching footsteps they dread hearing. It is largely in the nursing assistant's hands to make the residents' care experience satisfying, effective, and safe.

The preceding listing of a few of the things that caregivers are expected to do and the circumstances in which they do them should suggest that a calm, patient, and organized individual might be able to do a good job. The job also requires maturity and a professional attitude. If the facility has anything less than professional performance expectations of *all* the direct care staff, it is selling the quality of care short. Categorizing any direct caregiver as a nonprofessional or paraprofessional conveys the wrong message about those expectations.

Identifying the right *kind* of person to hire is a demanding task for any facility. Evaluating personality, attitudes, maturity, emotional stability, and capacity for professionalism before hiring a person is an inexact science. However, assessing the individual's job-related skill levels today is a little more precise than it may have been before OBRA.

OBRA set out to improve the quality of care for residents in long-term care facilities by improving the quality of the caregivers—from a skills perspective, anyway. All individuals working in nursing facilities (NFs) or skilled nursing facilities (SNFs) as nursing assistants or nurse aides either must have completed a training program and competency evaluation before their date of hire, or they must have completed the training before the date of hire and must complete the competency evaluation within four months of that date. Temporary or "agency" staff must meet the same competency standards. When an individual has completed the competency training and evaluation as required by the state, then the individual's name can be entered in the state nurse aid registry.

The training program must provide both classroom and "hands-on" training in clinical skills. The minimum classroom training time prior to any resident contact is 16 hours. That classroom training must cover the following subject matter.

1. Communication and interpersonal skills.

2. Infection control techniques (proper handwashing, handling of soiled linens, etc.).

3. Safety and emergency procedures, including the Heimlich maneuver.

4. Promoting residents' independence.

5. Respecting residents' rights.

The remainder of the required training time must include the following areas of instruction:

1. Basic nursing skills:

   ■ Caring for the terminally ill individual.

   ■ Measuring and recording height and weight.

   ■ Taking and recording vital signs.

   ■ Measuring and recording intake and output of food and fluids.

   ■ Caring for the resident's environment.

   ■ Recognizing and reporting abnormal changes in body functioning.

2. Personal care skills:

   ■ Bathing.

   ■ Grooming and oral care.

   ■ Dressing.

   ■ Toileting.

   ■ Assisting with eating and drinking.

   ■ Proper feeding techniques.

   ■ Skin care.

- Transfers, turning, and repositioning.

3. Mental health and social needs:

- Awareness of the developmental tasks of aging.

- Aide behaviors in response to resident behavior.

- Facilitating residents' free choice and dignity.

- Involving resident family for emotional support.

4. Care of cognitively impaired residents:

- Techniques for coping with the unique needs of individuals with dementia (Alzheimer's disease, Parkinson's disease, etc.).

- Communicating with cognitively impaired residents.

- Understanding behaviors of cognitively impaired individuals.

- Responding appropriately to behaviors.

- Methods to reduce the effects of cognitive impairment.

5. Basic restorative services:

- Training residents in self-care, based on their abilities.

- Use of assistive devices for walking, transferring, eating, and dressing.

- Maintenance of range of motion.

- Turning and positioning in bed and chair.

- Bowel and bladder training.

- Care and use of prosthetic and orthotic devices.

6. Residents' rights:

- Providing privacy and confidentiality.

- Promoting resident free choice and accommodation of needs.

- Assisting in resolution of grievances and disputes.

- Facilitating participation in resident and family groups and activities.

- Maintaining security for resident belongings.

- Promoting residents' right to be free from abuse, mistreatment, and neglect and the need to report any such treatment to appropriate facility staff.

- Avoiding the use of restraints in accordance with current professional standards.

All training programs, in order to be granted state approval, must meet the curriculum content requirements outlined above. As with hours over the required minimums, states are allowed to require more in curricular content, but they may not allow less. For example, the state may add the requirement that the program include training in cardiopulmonary resuscitation (CPR).

The OBRA legislation simplified the process of deciding what skills an applicant for a nursing assistant position should have by specifying the minimum content of a nurse aide training program. The minimum number of hours of training required, 75, is also specified. The states are free to approve longer, more comprehensive training programs, but they cannot approve any program that does not meet the minimum standard. Unfortunately, some of the longer, more comprehensive programs are being cut back to accommodate the minimums.

In addition to meeting the training requirements just described in order to be qualified to work in long-term care, the nurse aide staff must also keep their skills up through continuing education. This requirement calls for the nurse aide to complete at least 12 hours of continuing education per year. The facility must document this training and must evaluate the education needs of the staff so that training in areas of weakness can be provided.

Consumers need to be aware of what kind of training the direct care staff in long-term care facilities have had in order to have an idea of what they should be able to expect from their caregivers. For example, based on this training, consumers should be able to expect safe, thorough, and competent basic personal care. You should be able to expect protection of basic rights of privacy, dignity, and property and should have no fear of physical, verbal, or mental abuse. You should be able to expect quality care and quality of life, with no excuses.

It is important to understand that the direct care staff are sometimes too few in number in relation to the number of people in their care—even if the numbers look acceptable on paper. This can happen because of the higher level of acuity and greater care needs of individuals being admitted to long-term care facilities. More and more, care that was provided only in the acute care hospital setting in the past is being moved to the long-term care setting instead.

It is also important to understand how difficult the work really is: that it is both physically demanding and can be emotionally draining. As in most professions, complaints (often about uncontrollable problems) are heard far more frequently than praise for a job well done.

Consumers should have high expectations for the quality of care they or their loved ones receive in long-term care facilities and hold the facilities accountable for meeting those expectations. When your expectations are not met, raise the issue with the facility administration. If the facility meets or exceeds your expectations and the caregivers do a good job, a pat on the back is appreciated.

13

Recreation Therapy

HAVING FUN IN A LONG-TERM
CARE FACILITY

The bill of rights for residents in long-term care facilities discussed in chapter 7 guarantees residents the right to associate freely and to engage in activities that they enjoy. The facility has a role in assisting with fulfilling these rights by providing interesting things to do. Given the diversity of needs and interests in the mix of residents in the long-term care facility, this is no small order.

The recreation therapy program ("rec" therapy or "activities" in long-term care facility jargon) must be directed by a licensed or registered recreation therapist, a person who is eligible for certification by a recognized accreditation body, or an individual with at least two years experience in a social or recreation program in the past five years, one year of which had to be full-time in a patient activities program in a health care setting. An occupational therapist or occupational therapy assistant or an individual who has completed a training program approved by the state may also be considered qualified to lead the program.

The OBRA regulations specify the kind of training the recreation therapy staff must have, but at least as important as their training is their wit, humor, imagination, and patience. The recreation therapy function tends to be funded at minimal levels, reflecting an undervaluation of the importance of this function to residents. The positive impact of the program, however, can be determined by how much it adds to the residents' enjoyment of daily living. You cannot put a dollar value on a smiling face or the comment from a resident: "I like it here, there's something new to do each day."

Typically, the recreation therapy program will have a number of standard group activities such as musical entertainment, crafts, pet day, bingo, movie night, exercise (or "sittercise," which is targeted to people who are wheelchair-dependent), and parties for all birthdays and special occasions in the facility. These programs and many others led by the recreation therapy department can add tremendously to a resident's enjoyment of daily life.

In addition, the facility must take into consideration the physical, mental, and psychosocial needs of residents on an individual basis in developing a program that is designed to meet those needs as well. The facility is required to perform a comprehensive assessment of every resident's interests, past activities, and present mental and physical abilities and needs. Then the facility must develop activities that are of interest and value in meeting the resident's specific needs if existing program offerings do not. There are some possible indicators of poor recreation therapy program performance you should watch for:

1. Residents are often left sitting alone in hallways, dining hall, or their room, not talking or interacting with others, doing nothing.

2. Residents complain that "there's nothing to do here."

3. The posted activity schedule is frequently not followed, with planned activities being canceled or postponed, or it simply lacks variety and is limited in the number of activities offered and the frequency of activities. If the activity calendar is not posted in an area accessible to residents, inquire how the residents and staff are to keep track of what is happening, where, and when.

4. Family members are rarely involved in any activities-related programs.

5. Activities are not included in the care plan and there is no apparent link between the recreation therapy program and the rest of the care plan. The comprehensive assessment in the Minimum Data Set (section N, Activity Pursuit Patterns) is not used by the facility to help create an individualized recreation therapy plan for the resident.

6. The medical record does not indicate that outcomes are being evaluated in relation to the recreation therapy care plan.

7. The schedules for physical, occupational, or other therapies conflict with scheduled activities the resident has expressed an interest in and the facility makes no effort to resolve the problem to accommodate the resident's interests and needs.

There are many other things to look for, to be sure, and a problem with any of the items listed here does not necessarily mean there is a problem with the recreation therapy program as a whole. But if some of the things listed are present and as a consumer (resident or decision maker) you feel there is a problem, discuss it with the director of the recreation therapy or activities program.

14

Social Services

HELPING LIFE GO ON

Social services could aptly be called "life services." The social services staff in a long-term care facility can help immensely in the resident's quest to feel in control of her or his life again and to help that life go on. Social services can add greatly to the quality of a resident's life or create a void that can be very difficult to fill. The role of the social worker can vary by case. There are certain basic services that the social worker provides to each resident, but just as the nursing care plan must be customized to meet the assessed needs of the resident, the social services plan will need to be fitted to the resident's unique needs as well. In addition, the way each facility or organization defines the role of the social services department may influence the type of things the staff provide.

Both the quality and the qualifications of the person (many facilities have only *one*) or persons who occupy the role of the facility social worker affect how well this vital function is carried out. Stamina is a key factor, too. That is because the facility is required to have only one full-time, qualified social worker if the facility size is greater than 120 beds.

To meet the qualifications requirements in OBRA, the social worker must have a bachelor's degree in social work or a related human services field such as sociology, special education, rehabilitation counseling, or psychology and one year of supervised social work experience in a health care setting working directly with individuals, that is, not strictly in an administrative role [42 CFR Sec. 483.15(g)(3)(i)(ii)].

To help understand the role of the social worker in a long-term care facility, it is useful to know the definition of medically related social services used in OBRA:

> *Services provided by the facility's staff to assist residents in maintaining or improving their ability to manage their everyday physical, mental and psychosocial needs.*
>
> *[42 CFR Sec. 483.15(g)]*

At first glance, that may seem fairly simple. In practice, it can be a real load. Fulfilling this definition requires the social worker to be a strong resident advocate. Among the key roles social workers in long-term care may have are protection of residents' rights, prevention and detection of abuse, interventions in staff-to-resident/family problems, teaching staff about the fine points of resident self-determination, and encouraging facility practices and policies that promote resident independence, privacy, and dignity.

The social services staff may have primary responsibility for investigation of allegations of abuse, neglect, or misappropriation. They also are among the usual staff responsible for responding to episodes of crisis in the facility, be it a serious behavioral problem involving a resident, a personal crisis for an individual resident, or an emergency involving the entire facility. For this reason, social services staff should be *available* 24 hours a day. It is a good idea to discuss how the social services staff are reached after normal business hours, should the need arise.

Most of the duties of the social worker are not related to emergency or possible abuse situations. Some of the important actions the social worker may provide on a day-to-day basis relate to arranging medical or health-related services not necessarily provided by the physician, for example,

1. Arranging dental care, refitting or repair of dentures, and the like.

2. Arranging eye appointments and fitting of glasses.

3. Arranging hearing assessment and fitting of hearing aids.

4. Arranging podiatry services.

5. Arranging counseling services.

6. Arranging for the provision of special equipment or assistive devices.

7. Assisting with formulation of advance directives.

8. Arranging and coordinating clergy visits.

9. Assisting with the planning and provision of postdischarge care and support services.

10. Helping the resident and family or decision maker understand changes of condition in the care plan and assisting with discharge planning.

11. Providing information and support for decisions requiring informed consent.

12. Providing support for restraint and psychoactive drug reduction efforts.

13. Arranging transportation to appointments.

14. Securing clothing and other personal items.

15. Ensuring facility communication to family and decision makers.

16. Providing assistance with financial and legal matters, including assisting the resident or family member or decision maker to file a complaint about the facility.

17. Assisting the resident with orientation and adjustment to life in the facility and to its schedules, routines, and options that may be available to the resident.

18. Providing support to residents in distress and helping them cope with grief or loss.

19. Assisting with the management of problem behaviors.

20. Assisting with room or roommate changes and relations among residents.

21. Explaining facility policies and procedures and assisting the resident through the admission process.

The foregoing list is not inclusive and duties on it may be shared or handled completely by another facility department, such as nursing; some duties, for example, scheduling appointments and transportation, may be handled by the ward clerk or medical secretary on the resident's nursing unit. As a practical matter, it is useful to find out who handles the functions listed above, so that when there are needs to be met in each area or questions about appointments or policy, you know whom to talk to.

The social services staff must document their initial and on-going assessment of the resident and their interactions with each resident. The notes can be found in the medical record and are subject to the resident's and designated decision maker's right to review.

15

Hear My Voice

PRIVACY, DIGNITY, SELF-
DETERMINATION, PARTICIPATION,
AND ACCOMMODATION OF NEEDS

Your right to privacy and the assurance of your dignity are as fundamental and as intimate as the right to life itself. As important as these issues are, it is all too easy to find examples of these fundamental personal rights being compromised in the long-term care setting. Perhaps the reason for this is the ease with which violations of these rights can happen and the number of opportunities for violations to occur on a daily basis in a nursing home.

When you are living in your own home, protecting your privacy is something you do almost without thinking; in your own home, it is easy to do. In the long-term care setting, where residents are likely to share a room, protection of personal privacy is much more difficult and it is left entirely up to various staff members involved in your care.

Providing privacy on a daily basis and on the most personal level falls to the caregivers. Nursing assistants and licensed nursing staff need to be keenly aware of the resident's right to privacy in all the care they provide. The details are important: staff must treat the resident's room as the resident's private residence and respect it the same way.

■

PROTECTING YOUR PRIVACY

Here are some things residents should expect all facility staff to do to respect the resident's right to privacy:

1. All staff should *knock* and ask permission before entering a resident's room, even if the door is open. This rule, though very simple, is perhaps the most frequently brushed aside. Facility staff often justify walking freely into residents rooms by arguing that knocking takes too much time. I have even heard the excuse that "the resident can't respond anyway." The fact is, knocking takes only seconds, it is the accepted standard of practice that staff are taught to follow in the course of their training, and a resident's condition never excuses lack of respect for privacy.

2. When facility staff are in the room rendering care, the staff must take appropriate steps to ensure the resident's privacy. These steps include

closing the room door *and* drawing the privacy curtain around the bed or area care is being given *and* drawing the drapes over the windows, if need be. These are the minimum steps that should happen before the resident is assisted with bathing, grooming, dressing, transferring from bed or chair, turning and repositioning, placing a bedpan, major dressing changes or wound care, or any other personal care or treatments for which the resident's body may be exposed.

3. For a resident who needs to be fed by a staff member and who receives meals in his or her room, the decision to require privacy during meals should be made by the resident, family, or decision maker.

4. For residents who require assistance to get up to the toilet, staff should provide privacy to the greatest extent possible. This can be difficult because resident safety is a paramount concern. A resident who is confused and very unsteady simply cannot be left alone sitting on a commode or toilet. In cases where safety is clearly an issue, privacy can be accommodated only to the extent possible.

5. When a resident is being transported down the halls of the facility in a wheelchair, geriatric chair, or any other conveyance, the resident should be wrapped or covered sufficiently if he or she is not fully clothed. This is a serious problem when a resident is being taken to or from a common shower or tub room that is not in or adjacent to the resident's room. A common practice among facility staff is to simply use a hospital gown or blanket over the resident as "quick on, quick off" wrap for the trip down the hall. The problem with this method is that all too often, the gown or blanket is simply too small or poorly placed to actually provide privacy, leaving the person's legs, buttocks, or upper body exposed. Moreover, most wheelchairs have a space between the bottom of the backrest and the seat. If an openbacked hospital gown used as a covering is not fully wrapped around the resident, or if a blanket is simply draped over the front of the chair, the resident may be exposed from the back of the chair. Preventing this is no more difficult than placing a blanket in the chair prior to the resident getting in the chair and wrap-

ping it around the resident's body. It is warmer and more comfortable than bare skin on a vinyl wheelchair seat any day.

6. Auditory privacy, which is equally important, can be even more difficult to ensure, especially if the resident has difficulty hearing, even with a hearing aid. Under such circumstances, explaining new treatments, medications, and conditions—very personal discussions—without compromising the privacy requirements can be difficult. If closing the resident's room door will not do the job, it may be necessary for the facility staff to ask the resident to move the discussion to a private office or meeting room.

7. Any facility's staff should demonstrate sensitivity to privacy needs during visiting hours in particular. Even though there is still all the usual work to do, and the pace rarely slows down for the staff, they must still respect the resident's privacy needs when entering a room to provide care. If care is required when visitors are in the room, it is fine for the staff to ask the visitors to step out so the care can be provided.

8. You have the right to privacy in written communications as well. This means the letters you may send and receive are *your* business and must remain unopened until you open them, unless you authorize someone in the facility to open them for you.

9. To the extent allowed by law, your medical and financial records in the facility's possession must remain confidential. The facility is not allowed to release any information from your records without your permission. This does not apply when your care is being transferred to another health care provider or the record release is required by law.

10. Unnecessary staff should not be present while personal care or treatment is being given. This means that casual conversation between staff members while a resident is receiving care from only one staff member and the other staff member is simply making conversation is not acceptable. If they do not need to be there during personal care, they should not be there.

SELF-DETERMINATION
AND PARTICIPATION

OBRA provides some specific protections for the rights of self-determination and participation. The guiding philosophy of these requirements is explained in the regulation:

> *The intent of this requirement is to specify that the facility must create an environment that is respectful of the right of each resident to exercise his or her autonomy regarding what the resident considers to be important facets of his or her life.*
>
> *[42 CFR 483.15(b)(c)]*

The heart of the regulation is clearly in the phrase "*the facility must create an environment that is respectful of the right of each resident to exercise his or her autonomy regarding what the resident considers to be important facets of his or her life.*" To meet this requirement, the facility must influence staff members so their actions allow the resident to retain control over things the resident considers important. The facets of life that quickly become important to many residents entering the long-term care facility are often things that may at first glance seem minor details of daily living. However, from the perspective of the person whose daily living is being affected, they are far from trivial. Later in this chapter, we look at a short list of some areas where trouble can arise with respect to this requirement.

A facility should teach its staff that the resident's priorities should be most important in daily decision making. If it is successful in instilling this attitude, it is likely the facility routinely complies with this requirement and has happier, more empowered residents and families as a result.

One way to get a feel for how much emphasis the facility places on resident self-determination and autonomy is to ask to see written policies on the subject. Ask what the facility teaches its staff about this, how often it is taught, and how the policies are enforced. Look for the language about this in the resident's bill of rights. The most direct method of checking the facility's performance on this is

to ask other residents and their family members how they feel about their experiences with the facility and its staff. If there is the feeling that the facility calls all the shots, it may be that the facility has missed the mark in spite of a sound staff education plan and appropriate materials on self-determination.

DIGNITY

Webster's defines dignity as the "the state or quality of being worthy of respect, honor, or esteem." I can't think of a more fitting description of how residents in long-term care facilities deserve to be treated. Young or old, this definition does not change, and neither should the treatment of residents.

Just as the daily routine in a long-term care facility is fraught with opportunities for mistakes to be made resulting in violations of the right to privacy, so, too, can it be prone to indignities in residents' daily lives. In saying this, I refer to some actions that may under other circumstances be considered harmless or quaint and may occur without any intent to submit the person to any indignity. However, the rules are designed to prevent these subtle infringements of individual dignity just as decisively as they are designed to prevent deliberate or malicious indignities that may also constitute abuse.

Dignity issues in the long-term care setting often are linked to the little things that mean a lot in a person's day-to-day life. Some common dignity issues in long-term care facilities include:

1. Residents being addressed by pet names that they did not choose or give permission for. "Honey," "dearie," or "Grampa," among others, may not suit the resident and should not be used unless the resident allows it.

2. Residents dressed inappropriately or in clothing not chosen by the resident, when the resident is able to choose. Being left in a robe or hospital gown all day is not acceptable unless there is a medical reason for it or the resident makes the choice to be dressed that way.

3. Residents not being bathed and groomed or having hair styled and cut against their wishes. Residents left sitting in a hallway with food spilled on their clothing, a filthy bib on, or hair left ungroomed are deprived of their dignity and reflect shoddy care. Men should be shaved (if they customarily shave) and women should be groomed, including makeup if they desire it.

4. Residents being spoken to in "baby talk." Even if a resident is cognitively impaired, this is rarely appropriate or necessary. Adult residents should be spoken to as adults. This does not mean they cannot be spoken to softly, calmly, compassionately, or in a way that provides reassurance.

5. Residents not given the choice of their own tablemates at meals but this being dictated by the facility. To the extent possible, residents should be able to socialize with other residents of their own choosing.

6. Residents who are able to eat on their own, albeit slowly, not being allowed to do so. The resident should not be fed by staff simply because it is faster, and the resident should not be rushed at mealtime. Are residents who need to have assistance with eating always seated with other residents who need assistance for the convenience of the facility?

7. Residents not allowed to decide what activities in the facility they do and do not attend. When they express a desire to go to an activity and they need the facility staff's assistance to get there, it must be provided.

8. Individual activities not being under the resident's control. Residents should be free to watch television, listen to the radio, or read free of interference to the extent that they do not infringe on any other resident's rights.

9. Residents not given the freedom to control their daily schedule—the time they get up each day, when and how they bathe, and when they go to bed at night. Some regimentation and scheduling have to happen in a long-term care facility, but inflexibility on all issues of daily life is never necessary in order for the facility to operate efficiently.

10. For residents who are unable to respond to verbal communication, being spoken *over* or *about* rather than being spoken *to* when possible. It is an unwitting indignity inflicted by poorly trained staff, but it is an indignity to a resident when staff speak about the resident in the resident's presence as though he or she was not even there. While it may be true the resident cannot respond to what is being said, it is often true the resident *can* hear and may well understand what is being said.

There are many other affronts that may seem small or even insignificant in the flow of day-to-day living in a facility that can steal a person's dignity and individuality a small piece at a time. Preventing this from happening is the facility's responsibility and it requires a well-trained staff. It requires the staff to be sensitive to dignity issues in all the care they provide. It requires an ongoing education program by the facility on the issues of residents' rights, dignity, and privacy issues. Finally, it takes vigilance by the facility staff and administration and by informed consumers. When you feel there is a problem, voice a grievance to the facility at once.

■

PARTICIPATION: RESIDENT OR FAMILY COUNCIL

The right to participate in a resident or family council or group is an affirmation of the resident's rights as a citizen. The right to associate and assemble with others who have common interests is guaranteed by the First Amendment and the Code of Federal Regulations [42 CFR Sec. 483.15(c)].

A resident council or resident–family group or committee within a long-term care facility can be an effective voice for change in the facility and in the lives of the residents. OBRA does not *require* that there be a resident council or committee in a facility. What it does require of the facility is that any effort by residents or families to organize such a group or council be allowed to proceed without interference. The facility is also required to provide both space and privacy for the group to hold its meetings and the facility must designate at least one staff member to support the group's efforts and to provide responses to any issues that the group may raise.

The facility is neither required to take action on every issue that such a council or committee may raise nor obligated to accept each recommendation the group may present. The facility *does* owe the group due consideration of their concerns and recommendations and responses to them, generally in writing. The facility must also take the committee's requests and recommendations into consideration when formulating policy and making decisions about facility operations that affect residents' quality of life and quality of care.

A reputable facility will have no problem with the presence of an active resident council or committee. In fact, a wisely run facility will encourage such a development, simply because such a group can help to bring to light problems the facility may not otherwise know about and should act to solve. In addition, the group can be a great catalyst for self-directed resident group activities such as bazaars, group outings, social events in the building, and fund raisers for recreational equipment, books, and videos.

Facilities will often assign a social services staff member or member of the activities staff to be the designated staff person to work with the group and help with arrangements for their meetings. Though it is not required, the facility may provide regular reports to the committee about planned changes or improvements, not just responses to complaints or issues raised by the committee. Introducing new staff to the committee, describing new policies, or announcing other changes or additions to the facility or its services enhances the committee's place in the facility and gives the residents a greater sense of involvement.

The right to participate in other groups and activities, both inside and outside the facility, is included in this section of the regulations. Of particular importance are the person's interests and affiliations that existed *before* they became residents of the facility. To the greatest extent possible, a resident who wishes to continue participating in community groups and functions and religious activities must be supported by the facility. While the facility cannot be compelled to pay for or provide transportation to such functions, it must assist with making arrangements for such outings and must not interfere with such participation unless there is a medical reason for concern.

■
ACCOMMODATION OF NEEDS AND RESIDENT PREFERENCES

This requirement can be hard to quantify or describe in terms of when a facility has truly succeeded or failed to comply. The Interpretive Guidelines found in OBRA that give state surveyors direction on how to measure this describe **accommodation of needs** as "the facility's efforts to individualize the resident's environment."

What it really comes down to is how willing the facility is to allow the resident and family to individualize the resident's environment. Can residents put up wall hangings, memorabilia, and pictures in their room? What items of personal furniture and the like are allowed? If restrictions on these items exist, how reasonable and flexible are the restrictions? Do they really allow for expression of individual tastes and preferences?

The answer to some of these questions can be found in facility policy. If you or your family or decision makers are shopping around for a nursing facility, ask for facility policies on this. Do the same at the time of admission if you have not had the chance to do any advance planning.

Some facilities may be unduly restrictive or inflexible on relatively minor things, but most will be reasonable if you compromise a little. However, if they allow virtually no personal furniture, decorations, memorabilia, blankets, and the like, to be present in the resident's own room and they compel a resident to do, wear, eat, and drink virtually everything as presented by the facility with a general disregard for the resident's preferences, it is likely they are not in compliance with this requirement. They also have institutionalized an affront to their residents' dignity. Trouble can arise in several common areas:

1. The facility dictates the type and timing of bathing; for example, the comprehensive assessment in the MDS indicates that the resident's past practice at home was to take a tub bath in the evening but the facility gets the resident up at 5:45 A.M. for a shower, even though the resident expresses the preference for an evening tub bath. Generally, there is no good reason not to accommodate the resident's preference on this type of issue.

2. The facility rigidly dictates meal times. This is a potential problem area that seems to arise most often surrounding very early serving times for breakfast. Some facilities try to have their night shift staff get individuals up for breakfast prior to the start of the day shift. This can lead to the lightly staffed night shift having to get residents up long before breakfast is served so that they will have time to assist all those who need help getting up. While some people are early risers and may actually prefer being up early, those who do not may feel strongly that they would like more control over the time they get up. OBRA says they should have it. It should be possible to work with the facility to arrange somewhat later meal time and time arising.

3. The facility rigidly dictates times when residents who are dependent for care go to bed. In some facilities, staffing patterns are more influential over this issue than the resident's preference or right to choose. If the facility substantially reduces the number of staff in the building on the afternoon shift, remaining staff may start placing dependent residents in bed immediately after supper, whether they wish to be in bed or not. This, too, is contrary to the resident's right to choose and participate in decision making about care.

4. The facility's therapy department (if they provide it or contract for it) is allowed to schedule therapy times without regard to the resident's preferences or in such a way that the resident's meal times, social times, or activities are compromised in order to allow the therapy department to maximize the number of therapy units they do each day. Though therapy times are extremely important and there may be times when some scheduling conflicts will occur, there usually is a way for therapies to be scheduled with some degree of sensitivity to the resident's preferences and other activities.

These scheduling practices, left uncorrected, can lead residents to refuse to participate in the therapy sessions. This is not a good situation, since refusal to participate can jeopardize coverage for such services. If resident refusal to participate in therapy sessions is being caused by such invasions of the therapy schedule into other aspects of the resident's life, it is incumbent on the facility to address the problems with the schedule, not to simply threaten to withdraw the therapy.

5. The facility suddenly changes room or roommate. Advance notice must be given by the facility to the resident and/or the family or decision maker. There are times when a facility is placed in a difficult situation: called upon on very short notice to admit a person in dire need of the facility's services, the facility cannot do so without making some room assignment changes. The facility must do all it can to admit those in need, so it is beneficial for residents and facilities to try to cooperate on such situations.

6. The facility is not promoting the resident's independence to the greatest extent possible. This can become an issue when the facility staff continue to provide maximum assistance to a resident for eating, toileting, bathing, transfers to and from a chair, and walking (referred to as ambulation) when the resident should be doing these with "standby" assistance or supervision only. Why would the staff continue to do this as opposed to letting the resident do this independently? Speed. Facility staff are very busy and the shorter staffed the facility is, the busier they are. If residents can do these basic things themselves, but do them very slowly, the staff may be tempted to step in and just do it for them. For example, if a resident could actually be advanced to eating independently but the staff continues to feed the resident simply because it is faster, the resident's interests are not being served. Or if the resident should be walking using a walker but is more

often placed in a wheelchair and propelled by staff to meals, therapy, activities, and the like, simply because it is faster, again, the resident's best interests are not being served. In both of these examples, the resident's progress toward independence and discharge is actually likely to be slowed down.

The simple test to determine whether the facility is meeting the requirement for self-determination, dignity, and accommodation of needs is whether a person's needs and preferences are fully considered and responded to appropriately. This requirement is found in 42 CFR Sec. 483.15(e) of the regulations.

16

Saying "No" to Care

Your Right to Refuse

The right to refuse treatment is as personal a decision as you can make. It has implications that can involve more than the simple act of refusing to continue to receive care. It is an issue that can lead to concerns or even conflicts among family members, caregivers, and perhaps the community. OBRA provides some rules to protect an individual's right to maintain control over the decision to say "no more."

This issue hinges on whether you are your own decision maker, that is, whether you are considered competent to make legally valid treatment decisions. I will talk about the subject of decision makers and treatment planning in more detail in the next chapter on advance directives. For the purposes of this chapter, I will assume you are making your own treatment decisions.

With the exception of lifesaving emergency care, you must always be given the opportunity to express **informed consent** before treatment is given. Informed consent generally means that you have been given an explanation of the care to be provided, why it is necessary, what the expected benefits are, what the risks of treatment are, and who will be providing the care. For surgery and some other treatment methods, such as the use of physical restraints, consent must be expressed *in writing*. In the nursing facility setting, the right to refuse starts with the staff taking the time to *always* explain what care they would like to provide *before* they provide it. Even minor procedures, like checking a resident's pulse, taking blood pressure, or changing a small dressing, require that the staff explain what they are about to do, thus giving the resident the opportunity to say "no" or "not now, please."

Residents in long-term care facilities have the right to refuse even routine day-to-day procedures such as bathing, dressing, or eating. There may be times when a resident refuses to allow this type of care simply because of the facility's scheduling patterns. Or a resident may wish to refuse a given meal based simply on habits and preferences, and that's a right. The facility has the obligation to offer alternatives. The same holds true with medical care and treatments.

Refusing medical care—be it complex treatment or routine care—is not without consequences, and it is up to the facility to determine that residents who refuse treatment have been informed of the potential consequences of that refusal and that they understand them. The facility needs to find out why a resident refused treatment and attempt to address the problem, if there is one.

For example, if a resident refuses physical therapy after a hip replacement surgery, recovery is likely to be poor. The resident needs to understand the impact of the refusal on recovery and needs to be given reasons for reconsidering the refusal. If it comes to light that the resident often refuses to accept physical therapy because prescribed pain medication is not administered as ordered—prior to the therapy being given—then the resident has a valid reason to refuse and the facility has a problem to correct. The facility must inform residents of the consequences of refusal to allow care. It is very important that consequences be given careful consideration by the resident who is refusing or the decision maker who is refusing care to be given in the resident's behalf. The reasons for refusal should be discussed with the facility staff in order to give them a chance to address the reasons.

If a resident has an issue with a specific caregiver in the facility, not necessarily the care itself, the issue should be addressed in a private meeting with the nursing supervisor or director of nursing, or a member of the social services staff. An example of this type of problem is when the facility has male nursing assistant staff and a female resident strongly desires to have female caregivers only, at least for bathing. This arrangement can usually be accommodated.

When a resident refuses care or treatment, the facility must still meet the person's care needs. The facility must make the effort to identify care methods or alternatives that meet the resident's needs and gain the resident's approval. The inability of a resident to participate in care, such as physical therapy, must not be noted as a "refusal of care," which may occur at facilities that are running aggressive therapy programs. Under those circumstances, the facility's therapy schedule can be delayed when the resident is unable to perform the scheduled therapy in the allotted time. This throws the therapy schedule behind and may lead to the documentation of a "refusal" of therapy rather than documentation of a failure to meet goal progress or inability to perform the therapy due to pain, fatigue, or other reason that the facility may have been able to manage.

In addition to your right to refuse care, chapter 7, "Your Bill of Rights," also notes the right to refuse to participate in any experimental research. If the facility would like you to participate in any research project, particularly if it involves experimental medications or treatments, you must be informed of the nature of the research. You must be informed of possible consequences of your participation in the experiment and give your consent *before* the start of the project. Statistical studies that do not affect your care or treatment and do not involve the release of personally identifiable information about you as a subject of the research do not require your informed consent.

Perhaps the most important example of the refusal of treatment occurs when a person expresses the wish not to be kept alive by artificial or extraordinary means. A number of landmark legal cases involving this issue have been heard in the last 20 years and some important legislation has resulted from them in the past decade. In the next chapter, we will take a look at how OBRA and the Patient Self-Determination Act give consumers the ability to ensure that their health care wishes are carried out, even when they can no longer express those wishes themselves.

Advance Directives

TERMS OF EMPOWERMENT

Among the rules governing long-term care that ensure protection of your rights as a consumer of health care perhaps nothing is as important as the rules affecting your right to make decisions about your own care and treatment. There are some very specific protections on this issue, but they can be fairly complicated and, frankly, they are most useful if you know and act on them *before* you are incapacitated by a serious illness.

The federal Patient Self-Determination Act became law in December 1991. The law affects hospitals, nursing homes, home health agencies, hospices, and prepaid health care organizations. It established rules concerning your right to create what is known as an **advance directive,** that is, your express wishes, in written form, about whom you choose to make decisions concerning your care when you are unable to do so, and what types of care you may or may not wish to receive (see figure 4). The Patient Self-Determination Act requires the following:

1. That you be informed of your right to make health care decisions.

2. That you be informed in writing about how the facility will implement your rights and your advance directive.

3. That your medical record indicate whether you have created an advance directive.

4. That the facility will ensure compliance with any state laws on advance directives.

5. That the facility will act to educate its staff and the community about advance directives.

The definitions and rules that apply to the use of mechanisms for creating an advance directive vary from state to state. We discuss them in general terms here, but it will be necessary to find out what the rules are in your locality. Legal advice on creation of an advance directive is a very good idea.

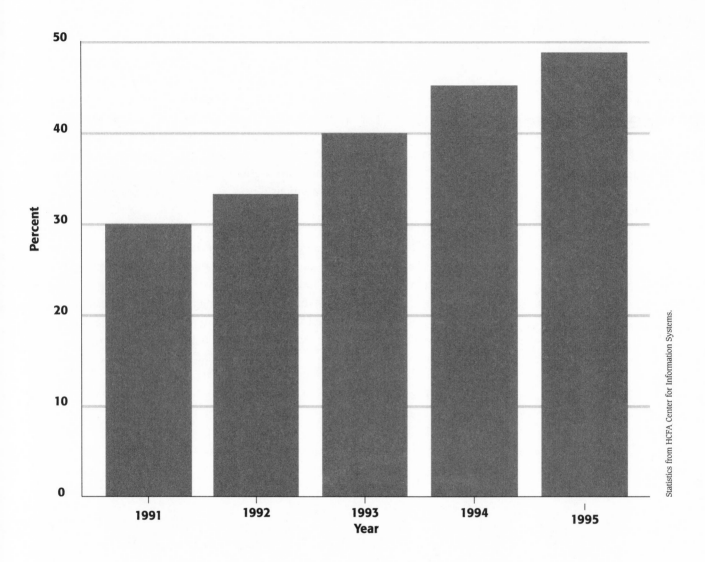

Statistics from HCFA Center for Information Systems.

Advance directives can help individuals in long-term care maintain control over their lives and the care and treatment they receive. The increase in popularity of advance directives as the result of OBRA is good news for consumers and caregivers alike, as long as the advance directives are appropriate for the individual and not simply a reflection of increased use of "do not resuscitate" directives. Prevalence increased from 30 percent in 1991 to nearly 50 percent in 1995.

INCAPACITY

The point at which a person's advance directive regarding a designated decision maker becomes activated is established by law. The regulations call for a process to make a medical determination in order to ensure that the person is truly incapable of making sound decisions; at that point the person can be considered *incapacitated.*

This is how a medical determination is completed to establish a person's capacity to make decisions:

1. An examination must be performed as prescribed by state law. Generally, it must be performed by a physician, a psychologist, or both.

2. OBRA does not specify methods or tests to be used for the evaluations, but they need to be appropriate to determine an individual's ability to comprehend information and make sound judgments and to determine whether the person has any cognitive (intellectual) impairments.

3. Each of the medical evaluations must be documented in the medical record.

4. The medical determinations must make a finding that the person is incapable of making decisions on treatment and/or finances before the advocate named in the advance directive has any authority to act.

5. The person who is the subject of the evaluation has the right to dispute the outcome of the medical determination.

Once this determination has been made, an agent previously selected becomes operative.

DURABLE POWER OF ATTORNEY

This document, known as a DPOA, enables you to designate someone you trust to handle financial and/or property matters for you in the event you become incapacitated. You may have this document written for you by an attorney or you may be able to obtain preprinted forms that are acceptable under your state's laws. Generally, this document confers *no authority* to make health care–related decisions. It is important for you to know your state's laws about what protections this document provides if you should choose to create a durable power of attorney.

You are the only one who can create a durable power of attorney document, and it must be done voluntarily, while you are competent to do so. You are also the only one who can revoke the document, and that would also have to take place while you are considered competent to do so.

There may be very specific legal requirements about this type of document, that relate to the following:

1. Language in the document.

2. Validity of the document.

3. Who witnesses the document and how it is witnessed.

4. Filing the document.

5. Effectiveness of copies.

6. Rules affecting the termination of the document.

7. Rules on resolution of disputes related to the document.

All things considered, even though preprinted forms for creating this document may be available, and there is no requirement that you use an attorney to create a durable power of attorney, it still may be a good idea to consult an attorney. The person you name to act in your behalf may be referred to as your "agent" or your "attorney-in-fact."

The person you designate must agree to do so and generally is required to do so in writing. It is wise to make sure the person you select understands exactly what you are asking before committing to the agreement.

DURABLE POWER OF ATTORNEY FOR HEALTH CARE

This document, called a DPOAHC, enables you to designate someone you trust to uphold your written health care or treatment instructions and/or to make those decisions for you in the event you become incapacitated. Unlike the durable power of attorney, this document generally does not confer authority over financial matters but does allow your agent to make health care decisions.

Neither the DPOA nor the DPOAHC becomes effective until *after* you have been deemed to be incapacitated. That is, the person you name in these documents has *no authority* to make decisions for you and *does not* become your decision maker or representative as soon as the documents are signed. You remain in control until you have been deemed incapable of making sound decisions by a process known as "medical determination" conducted by at least one physician and another practitioner, such as a physician or psychologist.

The person you name to act in your behalf may be referred to as your "advocate," "agent," "surrogate," "representative," or other term indicating that person's role in your care. It is very important to discuss your health care and treatment instructions with your advocate so that he or she knows your wishes clearly; you should then commit those wishes to writing as well. Here are some basics that apply to DPOA and DPOAHC:

1. These documents can be created only by you.

2. They must be created voluntarily.

3. They must be created while you are competent to make your own decisions.

4. Only you can revoke them, but your advocate may withdraw from that role as well.

5. They do not become effective (activated) until you are deemed incapacitated, or incapable of making your own decisions. The advocate has no authority to speak for you until the document is thus activated.

6. It generally is not necessary to have an attorney create these documents, but competent legal advice can be extremely valuable. Also, consulting with your physician about treatment options before committing your health care instructions to writing is an excellent idea.

CONSERVATORSHIP

This arrangement allows you to designate someone to assist you with managing your finances and property issues. You can create a conservatorship only while you are competent to do so voluntarily. The court appoints a conservator, officially empowering him or her to act in your behalf to pay bills and taxes and to buy, sell, or look after your property and the like as you direct.

You start the process to create a conservatorship by filing a petition with the court, nominating the person you wish to appoint. The court may hear testimony to determine that you are clear in your understanding of the action and may act to affirm or reject the nominee you have named, but the court may not name someone else instead. The court's order establishing a conservatorship will generally be specific in detailing the authority and responsibilities of the conservator.

In this arrangement, the conservator is accountable to the court, which may require the conservator to file reports with the court. Terminating a conservatorship will also require a trip to court, so it can be a fairly expensive option to use, but it can help get you the help you need, preserve some degree of control for you, and afford a degree of protection for your assets.

GUARDIANSHIP

A **guardian** is an individual appointed by the court to be your decision maker after the court has made finding that you are incapacitated. The court uses a process similar to a medical determination to establish whether a person needs to have a guardian appointed. The court may take testimony during a competency hearing to assist in making the determination about a person's incapacity. The person who is the subject of such a competency hearing has the right to be represented by legal counsel, call witnesses, and testify in his or her own behalf.

FULL GUARDIAN

A full guardianship generally confers sweeping authority to the person appointed: health care decision making, control of financial matters, and control of property including the right to dispose of it. While state laws governing the conduct of a guardian do afford protections to the ward (the person whose matters are being managed), there is the inherent disadvantage in the fact that you did not pick the person who can make some very important decisions— the court did.

The guardian is accountable to the court and is expected to act in your best interest. It is important to note that if the guardianship is established prior to the need for the ward to be placed in a long-term care facility, the law may place strict limitations on the guardian's ability to place the ward in a nursing home, particularly if there has been no period of hospitalization preceding the proposed admission. On the other hand, if the admission is required for protective placement, or if it is an involuntary commitment for treatment or for emergency detention, the law generally has specific provisions to allow placement in a long-term care facility, if only for a limited time to receive treatment.

Unfortunately, the need for the appointment of a guardian often arises in the case of a person who has been admitted to a nursing home after a serious illness when the person has not designated a decision maker. In this case, if there is no local family member or friend willing to assume the guardian role, the county social services department may be called on to recruit someone from the community. Needless to say, that places tremendous power in the hands of a total stranger.

In some jurisdictions, there may be certain restrictions on the powers of a guardian over the ward. For example, the guardian may not be allowed to establish an advance directive for a ward in terms of specifying types of medical treatment to be given or withheld. Another example relates to the use of psychoactive drugs (see chapter 20, "Powerful Stuff"). These drugs are used to alter mood or behavior, to promote sleep, or to treat a known mental illness. Some jurisdictions may not allow the guardian to give consent for the use of this class of drugs in the ward's care without a court order. Further, if the ward refuses to take the medications, the guardian may not give consent for the involuntary administration of the drug (such as crushing the pills and concealing it in food) even with a court order. In such circumstances, the law may require another step involving an involuntary commitment for mental health treatment before that type of drug administration can take place.

If you are likely to become a guardian for a family member, it is important to know the rules you are expected to follow. If the ward is in a nursing home, assistance may be available from the facility social services staff. For specific problems or when clear answers are not achieved, seek legal counsel.

The guardian for a person in a nursing facility is responsible for protecting the ward's rights, participating in the development of the ward's care plan, and giving informed consent for changes in medications or therapy and the use of any form of physical restraint. The facility must keep the guardian informed about any changes of condition or treatment of the ward. Care provided on an emergency basis (without advance consent) must be authorized with consent within 24 hours of the emergency care having been given. Following are some facts consumers and decision makers need to know about emergency changes to the care plan:

1. The guardian, decision maker, or resident must be notified of changes made on an emergency basis as soon as possible or within 24 hours.

2. Most emergency orders for things like physical restraints or the use of psychoactive drugs should be temporary and should be discontinued as soon as they are no longer needed. (Some states allow 12 hours to obtain consent.)

3. The facility needs to assess the cause of the problem leading to the emergency orders. This means a multidisciplinary team of the staff necessary must assess the problem and attempt to solve it.

LIMITED GUARDIAN

The court may appoint an individual strictly to oversee the ward's financial or property-related matters, conferring no authority to act on care and treatment decisions. This also may be referred to as a "guardian of the estate." The court may also decide to that a guardian with only care and treatment decision-making authority is appropriate and grant no authority over the ward's finances or property. This may be termed a "guardian of the person." These are both a form of a limited guardianship.

At first, the limited guardianship may seem to be a somewhat less complicated responsibility than the role of a full guardian, but for a guardian whose ward is in a nursing home, it can lead to some confusion on the part of the guardian and the facility's staff as to exactly what decisions the limited guardian can make. This is even more complicated when a given decision affects both health care decisions and the ward's financial resources.

For example, if the ward requires a medical test or procedure that is not covered by the ward's payer source, the cost then may be the responsibility of the ward's assets. This type of situation can be avoided if consumers create advance directives and designate decision makers.

GUARDIAN AD LITEM

This is generally an officer of the court, an attorney, who has been temporarily appointed by the court to act in the best interests of an individual who is incapacitated and facing protective placement who may or may not need a decision maker. Generally, guardians ad litem can recommend

care such as authorizing admission to a health care facility (hospital or nursing facility), but they usually cannot make health care decisions or create any form of advance directive. The guardian ad litem focuses on safeguarding the ward's rights and acts in the ward's best interests during court proceedings. The guardian ad litem also will make an independent report to the court.

■

LIVING WILL

A living will is a form of advance directive specifying the kind of care you wish to receive or not receive if you should become incapacitated. Not all states recognize a document called a "living will" but, in the absence of any other verifiable expression of your instructions, most health care providers and institutions will honor what you have put in writing, even if statutes do not specifically recognize this type of document.

Each state has rules for how advance directives must be created and witnessed, so check into the details to ensure it will operate the way you intend when the time comes. A living will made in conjunction with a durable power of attorney for health care properly executed and made a part of your medical record (as is required by law) *should* ensure that your care is carried out the way you want it to be.

■

UP IN THE AIR: WHAT HAPPENS WITHOUT AN ADVANCE DIRECTIVE?

There is no requirement for anyone to create an advance directive and no health care facility may lawfully require one as a condition for admission. No facility may discriminate against you in any way as a result of the presence or absence of an advance directive. Likewise, the facility may not transfer or discharge a person if the person chooses to refuse care unless the transfer is necessary to meet the person's care needs or the person's condition has improved to the point where the facility's services are no longer required.

Remember that the maker of an advance directive may revoke it at any time, as long as he or she is considered competent to do so. The maker of the advance directive may also modify it at any time and may withdraw and change the person chosen to be the advocate, but the person then chosen to be an advocate must agree to do so in writing. It is best to commit changes to writing, but some states allow such changes to be made by oral instructions.

When you create an advance directive, it is wise to place a copy with your advocate, a copy in a safe location that your advocate and/or family members have access to, a copy with your physician for addition to your clinic medical record, and a copy with your attorney, if you have one. To solicit the input of your physician and a competent attorney on your advance directive documents would certainly be an excellent idea.

You may choose not to create an advance directive. You certainly have that right, but what happens then? If you never lose your capacity to make your own decisions about health care and finances, it may not matter much. However, if you suffer health problems severe enough to incapacitate you, the many important decisions that you should make yourself will end up being made for you by someone else—possibly someone you would not have chosen.

In the absence of a specific, written directive from you to the contrary, the decision to do cardiopulmonary resuscitation (CPR), transfer to a hospital, and possibly place you on life support in the event you suffer a cardiac arrest may be made even if you would have opposed it. Some facilities may, in order to limit liability problems, follow the policy of providing all measures possible to preserve life in the absence of a known terminal illness. There are some steps you can take to avoid the delivery of such care if it is your wish not to have it:

1. Find out what facility policy is on provision of life-sustaining measures such as CPR and ambulance transfer to the emergency department.

2. Discuss your wishes with your doctor. If it is to have no resuscitation efforts by the use of CPR, convey

that to your physician and the facility in writing. For the facility to withhold life support, there must be a physician's order in your chart.

3. Create an advance directive such as a living will or other document that your state recognizes with comprehensive information about your medical treatment wishes.

■

MATTERS OF CONSCIENCE: WHAT ARE THE RIGHTS OF CAREGIVERS RELATED TO YOUR ADVANCE DIRECTIVE?

The rules that govern your right to make choices about your care and right to self-determination are strong, but at times the rights of caregivers may negate them. The health care facility (hospital, skilled nursing facility, nursing facility, home health agency, etc.) is not required to implement an advance directive to which it objects as a matter of conscience. The refusal to honor an advance directive on this basis must be allowed by state law and residents must be informed of the facility's policies in this regard at the time of admission. When you consider facilities, review their policies on advance directives carefully; if you have one or intend to create one, look for any potential conflicts between your directives and the policy. If there are any potential problems or questions, discuss them with the facility social services staff, the nursing staff, or the administrator.

A health care facility is not required to provide care that conflicts with a resident's advance directive. In other words, the facility cannot be required to provide care that may normally be expected of the facility in a given circumstance if the resident's advance directive specifically excludes it. To avoid any confusion over what the facility will do with respect to your advance directive, discuss your wishes and resolve any areas of confusion or conflict with facility policy in advance of the need for the facility to implement your directives.

18

Full Code, Slow Code, No Code

DECODING THE LINGO OF
LIFE SUPPORT

Once you have decided to create an advance directive, you will need to know some of the terms that are used to convey precisely your wishes to health care professionals. This chapter provides some insight on end-of-life care and decisions.

■

RESUSCITATION

The meaning of "resuscitation" depends on the nature of the person's condition, but this term is most often used in the context of the effort to revive a person whose breathing and/or pulse is absent. (You may hear of "fluid resuscitation," which is used in replacing critically needed body fluid volume, but generally this is not used in conjunction with immediate response to cardiac arrest.) Resuscitation usually refers to cardiopulmonary resuscitation, or CPR, which includes chest compressions to artificially support blood circulation when the heart has stopped beating (cardiac arrest) and artificial respiration, or rescue breathing, provided by mouth-to-mouth respiration or by the use of a mechanical ventilator or device called a bag-valve mask when breathing is absent.

The resuscitation situation where the heart has stopped beating is known as **cardiac arrest.** Whenever the heart stops beating, breathing also immediately stops. When this occurs it is imperative that resuscitation efforts begin immediately if the person is to have any chance for survival. Research has shown that the brain dies for lack of oxygen in as little as four to six minutes after the heart stops beating. This requires CPR to be effectively performed as quickly as possible after the cardiac arrest occurs.

There are also resuscitation situations where only rescue breathing is necessary because breathing has stopped while the heart continues to beat. This condition is known as **respiratory arrest.** In this case, it may be possible to sustain the heartbeat and prevent brain injury from lack of oxygen (hypoxia) if artificial respiration begins within a few minutes of the time breathing stopped. Depending on the cause of the respiratory arrest, it may be possible to sustain the person until breathing resumes. In some cases, it becomes necessary to place the person on a mechanical ventilator to sustain life.

In health care settings, these situations are commonly referred to as a "code," "code blue," or some other term that has been designated as a coded reference for such life-threatening emergencies. In an advance directive, if you indicate that you wish to have all lifesaving efforts performed in the event of cardiac or respiratory arrest, the term "full code" or simply "code" will be entered into your medical orders. When you have chosen not to have such measures performed, the term "no code" or "do not resuscitate" (sometimes called a DNR order) will be entered in your record. Also, in section A-10 of the Minimum Data Set the line indicating "do not resuscitate" will be checked. Each of these directives must be contained in your physician's orders.

The term "slow code" is sometimes applied to a resuscitation effort that limits the techniques employed and is therefore not a very aggressive form of resuscitation effort. There can be multiple reasons for taking this approach, but it generally is considered in the case of very ill, frail individuals of advanced age.

Under the best of circumstances, the likelihood of a cardiac resuscitation effort being successful is less than 40 percent in sustaining life; the likelihood of the resuscitated individual making a full recovery is far smaller, particularly among elderly individuals. You have the right to specify those measures you wish to have employed as well as those you do not want. This means you can elect to have emergency resuscitation performed in the event of cardiac arrest, but you may also decline to be kept alive on a ventilator. This could allow for the short-term use of a ventilator if your heartbeat is restored but call for it to be discontinued after a set period of time if there is no chance for recovery.

There are a number of techniques that go along with life support that you should be aware of. They are important to know about because it is possible to address them specifically in your advance directive. The more specific your advance directive's directions, the better. This information is presented because some techniques used in emergency life support situations are also useful in certain nonemergency situations. You may wish to exclude their use in the life support situation but not in other situations. If you happen to be incapacitated by the time the distinction has to be made, having your wishes in writing will be a benefit. The following techniques are useful in a number of medical circumstances, and your advance directive should indicate when you wish to have them administered:

1. **Endotracheal intubation** is the placement of a plastic device called an *endotracheal tube* in a person's airway (trachea), either orally or through a tracheotomy, to maintain an open passage to the lungs and protect the lungs from aspiration of fluids or vomitus during unconsciousness during surgery or during a resuscitation effort. A *nasotracheal tube* is inserted through the nasal passages (**nasotracheal intubation**) for the same purpose.

2. An **IV, or intravenous, line** is a plastic catheter that is inserted into a vein to establish an access to administer medications, nutrients, or fluids.

3. An **NG, or nasogastric, tube** is placed through the nose running down the esophagus to the stomach. It can be used to supply nutrients, medications, and fluids and to drain secretions or other fluids from the stomach.

4. A **ventilator, or "vent"** is a mechanical device used to breathe for patients whose breathing is too weak or absent. It can also be used to deliver higher concentrations of oxygen than room air contains.

5. A **cardiac monitor/defibrillator** is a device capable of measuring the heartbeat and electrical activity of the heart. The defibrillator can deliver an electrical shock to the patient useful in resuscitation efforts to try to restore the heart's normal rhythm.

The use of these and other techniques may have an impact on your advance directive. Other issues such as the continuance of hemodialysis may also be very important to consider with your physician in certain circumstances. In any case, it is a good idea to review your advance directive with respect to your care and treatment instructions with your doctor.

INTUBATION

Intubation is a very important step in the resuscitation process. Properly performed, it is a generally reliable way to maintain an open airway to the lungs that also protects the lungs from aspiration, or inhalation of vomitus or other fluids. It is usually performed as soon as possible after a resuscitation effort begins. The device used, the endotracheal (ET) tube, is also necessary when an individual is placed on a ventilator. For this reason, individuals who do not wish to have CPR performed or do not wish to be placed on a ventilator may indicate "no intubation," in an advance directive, especially if they are using a form that has that option printed on it.

That is fine as far as it goes, but other uses for intubation must not be ignored when the directive is created. Intubation can be necessary for some extremely important short-term uses that do not relate to the long-term use of a ventilator or the provision of CPR. For example, a severe allergic reaction to a new medication, food, or some other agent is treatable, but it can be fatal if the airway swells and becomes obstructed. Intubation can prevent a tragic outcome from a very treatable cause. Once medications are administered and the reaction abates, the endotracheal tube is removed.

To prevent any confusion regarding your preference on this technique, spell it out in your advance directive. If you do not wish intubation under any circumstances, state that. If you wish to exclude its use for long-term life support on a ventilator or for resuscitation purposes only, state that explicitly. If you do wish to have CPR and life support provided in the event of cardiac arrest, your directive should specifically allow the use of endotracheal or nasotracheal intubation.

INTRAVENOUS THERAPY

An IV, or intravenous line, is a section of tubing inserted (started) into a vein during a resuscitation effort to give direct access to the bloodstream for administration of medi-

cations or fluids. In some facilities, the choice of whether or not to have an IV placed is discussed as part of end-of-life decision making about resuscitation. However, an IV may be beneficial in situations that do not relate to resuscitation, for example, in administering fluids to reverse quickly the effects of dehydration caused by vomiting or diarrhea. IVs are also useful for the rapid administration of medications such as antihypertensive drugs (to treat critically high blood pressure) or certain antibiotics. Your advance directive should take such uses into account and specify whether you wish them to be allowed.

NASOGASTRIC TUBE

Placement of a nasogastric (NG) tube as part of a resuscitation effort is uncommon; it is usually done only if the abdomen is distended (enlarged), indicating that a lot of air has accumulated in the stomach, making ventilation less effective. The nasogastric tube is more common in the long-term life support situation, used for tube feeding and providing fluids and medications when the patient cannot swallow.

The NG tube is useful at other times as well, and it may be wise to consider those situations when formulating an advance directive. For example, an NG tube can be placed temporarily to remove stomach contents in the event of an accidental poisoning, or it can be used for tube feedings during recovery from oral, facial, or throat surgery or after facial injury. Use of an NG tube is also common during and after abdominal surgery and in the treatment of a bowel obstruction. If you wish to allow these short-term limited types of uses for an NG tube but do not want it to be used for long-term life support, you can specify that in your advance directive.

VENTILATOR

The decision regarding the use of a mechanical ventilator is generally linked to the issue of long-term life support when a person is in what is called a "persistent vegetative state" and unable to breathe independently. There are times, however, when the use of a ventilator is necessary for short, defined periods of time, such as a brief recovery period after a major surgery, but it is the first use mentioned that most individuals creating an advance directive tend to think of and generally wish to prevent.

Discussion of the use of a ventilator with your physician is useful to help you gain a clearer understanding of circumstances that may affect you and for guidance on what parameters you may wish to consider for the use of a ventilator in your advance directive.

■
CARDIAC
MONITOR/DEFIBRILLATOR

The use of the cardiac monitor/defibrillator in an emergency situation allows caregivers to follow the rate, rhythm, and electrical activity of the heart and identify abnormalities. The use of a cardiac monitor by itself does not constitute "artificial life support," though the device is an essential part of a resuscitation effort using what is known as "advanced cardiac life support." The use of a cardiac monitor is common in the acute care or hospital setting on a routine basis. Its use generally is not an issue that needs to be addressed in the advance directive.

The use of a defibrillator, which is an integral part of some models of cardiac monitor, is worth discussion here. The defibrillator consists of two paddles that act as electrodes for the cardiac monitor when simply placed against the chest. This allows the monitor to be used to evaluate the heart's electrical activity very quickly. The paddles also can be used to deliver an electrical shock to the heart in order to treat dangerous heart rhythms or to attempt to restore a heartbeat to a heart that has stopped beating.

The use of the defibrillator occurs in life-threatening situations but may not always occur in a resuscitation effort. The question of whether to allow the use of a defibrillator in the creation of your advance directive should take into account the use of the device in various situations. For individuals wishing to have no resuscitation, the DNR directive may

suggest to some clinicians that the use of a defibrillator is also not desired. However, since the defibrillator can be used to treat serious heart conditions before resuscitation is necessary, it is beneficial to consider these cases as well in the advance directive.

■
YOU CANNOT GET THERE FROM HERE: "DO NOT TRANSFER" ORDERS AND SUPPORTIVE CARE

The decision to transfer a resident from a long-term care facility to an acute care hospital for treatment of sudden illness or injury may seem to be automatic, but in fact, it is not. Many facilities will ask if such transfers are going to be desired and authorized by the resident or the resident's decision maker, especially when an advance directive containing the decision to decline resuscitation is on file.

Though it may seem logical to assume that a person with such an advance directive will not require transfer to a hospital emergency department for emergency life support, extending the idea of "no transfer" in all circumstances could be a mistake, yet unless the advance directive is specific on this point, the facility's staff *could* make that assumption.

There are a number of therapeutic and diagnostic services that can be provided in the hospital setting that can prevent serious complications of treatable conditions, ensure comfort, and correctly identify and treat the causes of a change of condition. In general, the decision to decline all transfers to a hospital for care and evaluation makes sense only in the case of a person who has established an advance directive and written physician's orders for no resuscitation (no code) and who has a known terminal illness where death is imminent. Otherwise, keeping the option for transfer to the hospital open for treatable conditions makes sense, especially if the facility's capabilities are limited where the needed services are concerned.

In some long-term care facilities, the term "supportive care" is used in conjunction with the "no code" advance directive. It is a good idea to find out what the facility means when it uses this term. In general, the phrase is used to describe care that includes basic nursing care such as bathing, dressing, hygiene, turning and repositioning, feeding and hydration, routine medications, skin care, and pain control. Services such as restorative and rehabilitative therapies, advanced nursing procedures, and life support interventions are generally not included.

Unless you know exactly what supportive care includes, it is a good idea to specify in your written advance directive the care you desire in an end-of-life circumstance. This will require the long-term care facility to meet the requirements *you* set—not its own.

19

Is This Pill Really Necessary?

Freedom from Unnecessary Drugs

The practice of medicine was once left pretty much in the hands of the doctor, particularly when it came to prescribing medications. In recent years, though, insurance companies, concerned practitioners, advocacy groups, and the government have increasingly emphasized modifying the practice of medicine. OBRA contains some very specific rules about the use of medications.

OBRA does not directly regulate the physician's conduct or prescribing practices. For example, the regulations do not establish government sanctions against the doctor for violating the rules. Instead, they penalize the long-term care facility if it allows the doctor to be out of compliance. This roundabout approach does have value in that it compels the nursing facility to be keenly aware of the medications each resident is taking, the dosage, and the reason for the medication to be given. It also compels the facility staff to be aware of the potential side effects of each medication, the desired therapeutic effects, and potential interactions with other medications the person is receiving. Finally, the system compels the facility staff to ensure proper informed consent is obtained and to play the role of the resident advocate where the use of medications is concerned.

■ ROLES OF YOUR PHYSICIAN AND THE CARE FACILITY

By law, a health care consumer or decision maker is allowed to hold both the physician and the facility accountable for appropriate prescription of medications. The role of the physician is to determine the need for the medication based on the patient's condition and write an appropriate order that includes the correct drug name, dose, route of administration, time of administration, and in some cases when to withhold the drug or give a different dose (parameters, as they are called). The role of the facility is to make sure that the order is obtained and clearly understood, that it is explained to the resident and/or decision maker, in some circumstances obtain written consent for the administration of the drug, and, finally, after those steps are completed, administer the medications safely. In the case of residents who self-administer drugs, the facility still is responsible for ensuring safe, timely, and accurate medication administration.

The goal of the rules against *unnecessary* drugs is pretty clear whether you have a medical background or not: it simply requires that the doctor and the facility must each act to ensure that no medication is given without a diagnosis or symptom that the drug is intended to treat.

Once the order is written, and the medication is being given, the nursing staff must know what potential problems it can cause and observe for signs and symptoms of those problems. They must know the appropriate dose, the right route of administration, the dose timing, whether the medication can be crushed (some medications should not be crushed) if necessary to make it easier to swallow, and if the medication should or should not be given with food. The nursing staff must be on the alert for signs of drug side effects, overdose, toxicity, interactions, and allergic reactions. The nursing staff must verify that the doctor's orders are correct and appropriate for the drug that has been ordered. The facility staff ultimately is responsible for ensuring that the medications the doctor has ordered are necessary to treat the resident's condition or symptoms. They are also responsible for the documentation of effects of the drugs—both desired therapeutic effects and the undesired side effects that occur and, of course, the fact that the medication has not been effective in any way at all. The following checklist will help guide your questions about medications being used in care and treatment:

1. What is the reason for the medication (diagnosis)?

2. What is the name, dosage, route of administration, and timing of the medication?

3. Why is it necessary? What is the expected benefit in treating a condition?

4. What alternatives have been tried and are there others that could be tried?

5. What are the possible side effects, adverse reactions, and interactions with other medications?

6. How will the facility monitor whether the therapy is working or causing more problems?

7. Will the dose be reduced over time, increased, or stopped? Does the body build up tolerance to the drug, making it less effective over time?

8. Is the medication actually prescribed to treat the symptoms of side effects of other drugs?

9. Can residents self-administer the medication?

10. Does the medication duplicate a drug that is already being given?

11. Is the drug being ordered a name brand drug or is it a generic substitute?

The next chapter, "Powerful Stuff: Rules That Protect You from Misuse of Psychoactive Medications," discusses what you need to know about the category of medications that helped instigate the OBRA regulations in the first place. Despite rules intended to drive down the use of psychoactive medications in nursing facilities, their use has continued to increase. Consumers need to be aware of this category of medications and how they should be managed.

■

ROLE OF THE CONSULTANT PHARMACIST

OBRA requires that facilities obtain the services of a licensed pharmacist to do the following:

1. Advise on all aspects of the provision of pharmacy services in the facility.

2. Establish a system for the tracking and accounting for controlled substances.

3. Review the drug regimen of each resident at least once a month and report any irregularities to the attending physician and the director of nursing.

The last of these roles is of particular importance to consumers. The consultant pharmacist performs a vital function in making sure that the medications ordered by the physician are appropriate, do not interact with other medications the person is taking, are not likely to cause allergic reactions, do not duplicate the functions of other drugs the person is taking, are not being given to counteract side effects of other drugs, are ordered in appropriate doses, and are administered by the correct route and timing. To do this the pharmacist must evaluate the following:

1. Each medication for an appropriate medical indication (diagnosis) and watches for so-called off-label uses. Off-label uses are prescriptions written to use a drug for a condition that is not included in the manufacturer's list of intended uses.

2. The known interactions among the drugs each resident is receiving. Interactions are the adverse or undesirable effects that can be caused by drugs that react when they are given together.

3. The known allergies of each person and the likelihood the medications the doctor has ordered will trigger an allergic reaction.

4. The diagnosis for each drug being given to determine whether multiple drugs are being given for the same purpose (polypharmacy). There are times when it is necessary to use more than one medication to treat the same condition, but it is important to make sure that this is the case when multiple medications are being used to treat the same condition. This problem can occur when more than one doctor is caring for a person and the doctors do not communicate with each other as medication changes are made.

5. The dose, schedule, and route of administration for each drug to make sure each is correct for each medication and individual case.

In addition, the facility is responsible for ensuring that drugs are accurately received and administered, properly and securely stored, and accurately labeled in order to prevent improper drugs, inaccurate dosages, and administration of medications to the wrong person, by the wrong route, or at the wrong time.

Typically, families and consumers do not get a chance to talk directly to the consultant pharmacist, who often is a private contractor in the facility only for a day or two each month and generally does not sit in on care planning conferences. This does not mean consumers, family members, and decision makers are not entitled to timely answers to their questions or concerns on medication issues. If you have concerns or questions, you should raise them with the facility staff and, if necessary, they can share the consultant pharmacist's insights with you in the form of the reports that he or she files or they can contact the pharmacist by phone. You also should consult with the physician or, if you have a pharmacist whom you have dealt with in the past, with that pharmacist as well.

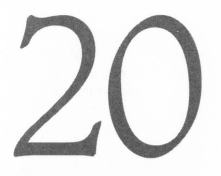

Powerful Stuff

THE RULES THAT PROTECT
YOU FROM MISUSE OF
PSYCHOACTIVE MEDICATIONS

As we saw in the chapter on unnecessary drugs, several factors must be considered any time medication is being used as a part of the care plan. The list gets even longer when the drugs are in a category known as **psychoactive drugs**—drugs that alter mental processes. Since the number of nursing home residents being treated for psychiatric diagnoses has been steadily increasing (see figure 5), we discuss this often controversial subject in some detail here.

Psychoactive medications may be compared, in some ways, to an automobile. Used properly, each can be safe, effective, and tremendously beneficial to the person's quality of life. But they must be used for the right reasons, under the control of someone who thoroughly understands their workings and hazards. Take away the control, understanding, and proper use and these drugs, like automobiles, have the potential to cause serious problems.

Despite the risks some of these medications carry, they have a legitimate place in long-term care. They can be very effective in treating psychotic behavior, schizophrenia, schizoaffective disorder, delusional behavior, Tourette's syndrome, Huntington's chorea, and some forms of dementia. Medications used to treat these conditions usually are in a category known as **antipsychotic** drugs.

Other drugs included in the category of psychoactive medications are used to treat anxiety disorder, panic disorder, and organic mental disorders (also referred to as organ brain disease), which includes a variety of cognitive disorders such as delirium, dementia, and amnesia. Drugs used to treat these conditions or their symptoms fall into a general category called **anxiolytic** or **sedative** drugs. These agents may be used to treat severe agitation, aggressive behavior, and sleep disturbances.

Included in the category of anxiolytic (antianxiety) medications is a family of drugs known as **benzodiazepines.** Over the years, their use for behavioral management in long-term care became quite common; indeed, they were typically prescribed for a wide variety of "problem behaviors," which in many cases should not have required these drugs. This trend and the fact that these drugs have been implicated as the cause of other problems, such as falls, decline in functional (self-care) status, worsening mental status, side effects, and the possibility of dependency, have led to stringent guidelines for their use in the long-term care regulations.

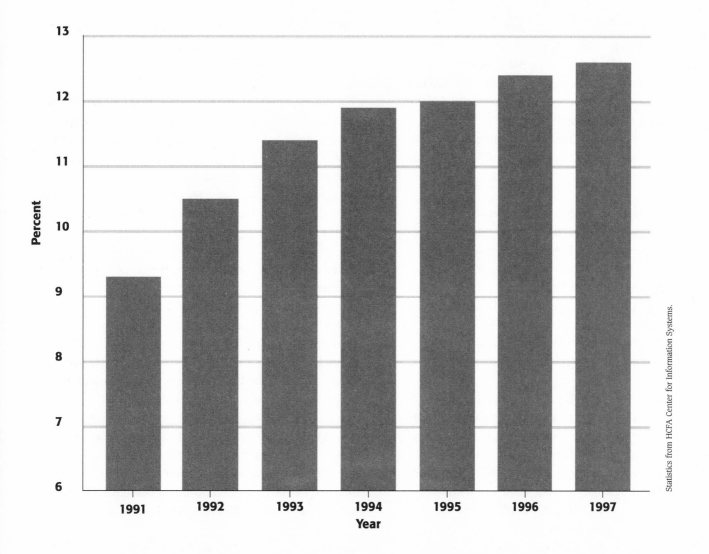

Statistics from HCFA Center for Information Systems.

One of the specific goals of the OBRA nursing home reforms was to prevent individuals with mental illness from being placed in nursing homes unless they had physical care needs that justified the placement. The regulations include what is known as PASARR screening (Preadmission Screening/Annual Resident Review) to accomplish this goal. Despite this process, the number of nursing home residents reported with a psychiatric diagnosis increased from 9.3 percent in 1991 to 12.6 percent in 1997.

There are two groupings of benzodiazepines available: short acting and long acting. The rules do not prohibit the use of these drugs, but they do restrict the dosages, reasons, and length of time the drugs can be used and establish criteria for limited exceptions to the guidelines. The use of long-acting benzodiazepines for behavior, not to treat seizures or as a muscle relaxant, is restricted to situations where short-acting benzodiazepines have been tried and have failed, the dose is within the limits stated in the regulations, causes of the behavior have been assessed, and the drug proves to be beneficial in maintaining or improving the resident's ability to function.

Drugs used to treat depression—**antidepressants**—are also in the category of psychoactive medications and are included in the regulations. There have been studies that indicate that the prevalence of major depression among individuals in long-term care facilities may exceed 20 percent of the total population. The number of individuals suffering with less severe situational depression may approach 50 percent of those in long-term care facilities, particularly among those individuals recently admitted.

The prevalence of depression, its profound impact on the individual's quality of life, and the ability of modern therapies to effectively treat depression have led to the creation of rules governing the use of antidepressants that are slightly more liberal than those applied to other categories of psychoactive drugs. For example, the use of written behavioral monitoring record systems, a requirement for most other categories, is not necessary when depression is diagnosed, thus eliminating the burden of paperwork, which sometimes discourages caregivers from treating depression.

Also, unlike the guidelines for the other categories of psychoactive drugs, the regulations do not specify daily maximum doses or time limits for antidepressant agents.

■
"PROBLEM BEHAVIORS"
DEFINED

Psychoactive medications usually are prescribed when the resident exhibits behaviors that are of concern to the facility, physician, family, or, as is often the case, all of the above (see figure 6). Antisocial, aggressive, bizarre, or inappropriate behavior of one type or another may be considered "problem behavior" and if it is recurrent or ongoing and nonmedication interventions do not help, the use of a psychoactive medication may be considered.

Back in the days before OBRA, such behaviors would lead to a fairly common response: calling the physician and asking for an order for "something to settle the resident down" or to "help the resident relax." All too often, the doctor simply complied and, even with the best intentions to use the medications on a temporary basis until the crisis passed, the orders frequently became a fixture, used far longer than necessary.

Given on a routine basis, at dosage levels appropriate to an emergency situation, these drugs might well leave the resident in a stupor: groggy, lethargic, unsteady, even unable to walk. Such conditions were then attributed incorrectly to the resident's "declining condition" or "advancing age." A resident in such a condition is easier to provide care for than a resident who is combative or abusive to staff or other residents. Eventually, side effects might further debilitate the resident, causing genuine physical decline and devastation of the resident's quality of life. Through all of this, it was not uncommon for assessment of the cause of the behavior that led to the medication's being ordered in the first place to be overlooked. OBRA is designed to prevent this unhappy course of events from occurring.

Behaviors that can fall into the problem behavior category can cover a wide range of type and severity. The fact is, the *behavior* is generally not really the problem; the behavior is a symptom of the real problem. In most cases, treating the real problem will also eliminate the behavior. Since that will often involve solving a problem that does not require the use of psychoactive medications, that is the mandatory first step: a thorough assessment to determine the *cause* of the behavior.

In cases where a psychiatric evaluation has been done and a mental disorder is diagnosed that is appropriate for treatment by the use of a psychoactive medication, there is still the need to assess other factors that may trigger the

■

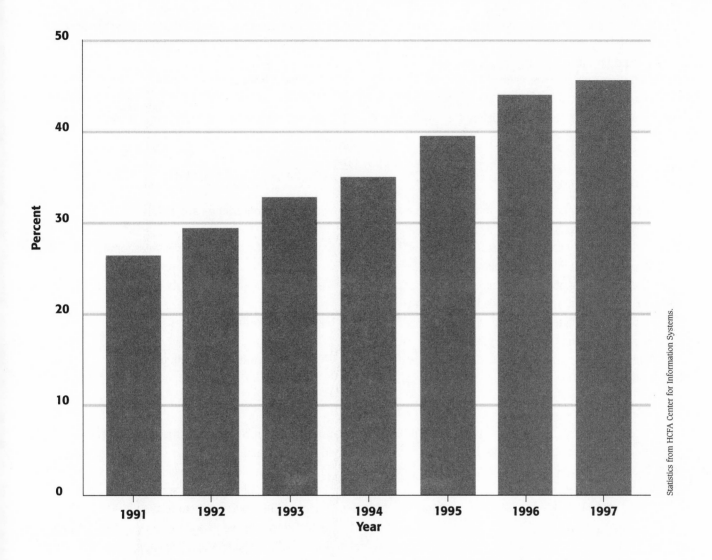

Statistics from HCFA Center for Information Systems.

Despite the very specific restrictions designed to limit the use of psychoactive medications, their use has increased nationwide from 26.4 percent in 1991 to 45.6 percent in 1997. The stringently regulated antipsychotic medications were in use on 17 percent of the nation's nursing home residents in 1997. Increased use of antidepressants may also have contributed to the increase in these medications.

behavior. In that case, the diagnosis may justify the use of the medication, but even then the facility and the doctor must continue to reduce or eliminate the use of the drugs, unless such efforts are clinically contraindicated, by continuing to assess the resident's behavior and by trying to find alternative treatment methods. This holds true even for individuals who have a history of mental illness prior to their admission to the long-term care facility and who had been taking psychoactive medications before they were admitted to the facility.

AGGRESSION OR ABUSIVE BEHAVIOR

Topping the list of problem behaviors likely to trigger the use of psychoactive medications is physical aggression on the part of a resident toward caregivers, visitors, or other residents. Striking out, biting, kicking, grabbing, pinching, spitting, scratching, throwing objects, and making threatening gestures or verbal threats will all be likely to prompt a response from the facility. Often these behaviors are accompanied by verbal outbursts: name calling, swearing, screaming, crying, or making graphic or sexually oriented abusive comments.

As extreme as these behaviors may seem, they rarely are the result of a mental illness. More often, they are the result of anger, frustration, fear, or pain that cannot be expressed if the resident is also unable to communicate as the result of brain damage from a stroke or a dementing illness such as Alzheimer's disease, Pick's disease, or Huntington's chorea.

Identifying the source of the behavior can often be as simple as meeting some basic need: eliminating noise, drawing the drapes, getting a glass of water, changing position, getting to the toilet, adding or taking off a blanket. Preventing an "agitated," confused resident from grabbing or pinching caregivers or other residents may be accomplished by supplying a doll or soft pillow to hold. It is incumbent on the facility to be alert for indicators of what triggers problem behaviors and to be imaginative in finding solutions that protect not only the other residents but the "problem" resident as well.

DEPRESSION

High on the list of behaviors that are worrisome among long-term care residents are the signs and symptoms of depression:

1. Withdrawal from usual activities.

2. Lack of interest in hobbies, bathing, dressing, and grooming.

3. Loss of appetite and weight loss.

4. Withdrawal from friends and family.

5. Expressions of sadness, hopelessness, or anxiety.

6. Chronic fatigue and/or inability to concentrate.

7. Loss of self-worth.

8. Wishing for death or even talk of suicide.

9. Alcohol abuse.

Because depression can have such a profound effect on an individual whose ability to recover may be impaired by advanced age or multiple physical health problems, the facility must be diligent in observing for signs and symptoms of depression and in reporting them to the physician. This is particularly true in the period immediately after admission to the facility, when people are confronted with many changes that they may feel powerless to control. They suffer the loss of control, loss of health, and loss of privacy; they may fear loss of home and finances; they experience loss of contact with spouse, family, and friends. It is no surprise a condition referred to as **situational depression** may develop during this difficult time.

A resident may face events that loom larger than they really are, perhaps even overshadowing health problems and overwhelming coping mechanisms of the individual. For example, a resident may be concerned about a spouse living alone at home, especially if the partner at home has been largely dependent on the resident for many daily functions.

Concern over finances and how care will be paid for can cause anxiety and confusion despite the best explanations of the options available by the social services staff. Simple things can add tremendous weight to the burdens of ill health: Who will pay the bills? Who will take care of my pets? Who will take care of my house?

The sudden change from independence in one's own home to partial or total dependence in a communal living setting can impose a tremendous sense of loss: loss of self-determination, loss of control, loss of self-worth, and loss of dignity. The losses of companionship of spouse, family, and friends can impose a sense of isolation and loneliness.

Financial and household concerns can be allayed by planning ahead, but in most cases the need for care arises so suddenly that planning simply has not been done. Instead, everything is dumped on the ill person, his or her family, and friends when one dizzying spell of illness leaves only a few days to try to get things organized. The person may be moved from emergency care in an ambulance to the hospital to the subacute care or swing bed unit to the rehabilitation center to the nursing home in a period of a few days. Through all of this, there are forms to fill out, papers to read, documents to sign, consents that must be given. The ill person can easily become bewildered by it, feel overwhelmed, and sink into a sense of hopelessness. The nursing facility is responsible to help identify and deal with the circumstances that can lead to this situation. Nursing and social services staff together with the attending physician must act to help the resident and family or decision maker to sort it all out and arrive at a plan that creates a sense of order and empowerment.

The physician must do an assessment, which includes conferring with nursing and social services staff or reviewing their notes to determine if additional medical interventions are necessary. This assessment of what is known as "psychosocial adjustment" is a mandatory part of the detailed assessment process in the federally specified assessment document called the Minimum Data Set, or MDS (discussed in chapter 9). The physician and the facility have specific guidelines to follow in meeting the requirements of the assessment process in regard to psychosocial adjustment and depression.

SLEEP PATTERN DISTURBANCE

A common problem of concern in the long-term care facility is insomnia, or the inability to achieve a "normal" sleep pattern. Insomnia can be part of the symptoms caused by several different problems or it may arise as a direct result of the unfamiliarity and disruptions of the nursing facility itself. In addition, it is possible that the sleep pattern that is normal for the individual is considered abnormal by the facility staff. OBRA attempts to prevent this from occurring by making assessment of the person's customary sleep habits a part of the MDS (Section AC-1, Customary Routine). However, if the facility does not accurately use the assessment tool or fails to utilize the information gained by it, the resident's normal sleep cycle may be misinterpreted as a problem.

If that occurs, the facility staff may report to the physician that the resident is "restless" or "wanders late into the night," which may result in an order for sleep-inducing medication to deal with the problem with little further assessment. This situation could occur even though the facility should have known from its MDS assessment that the resident's normal time to go to bed at home was late at night rather than 8:30 P.M., when the facility staff customarily put residents to bed. Before medication to treat such an apparent sleep pattern disturbance is considered, the physician must document an assessment of the possible causes, which should include the MDS information about the person's sleep habits in the past. Causes for an apparent sleep pattern change that do not require drug treatment should be ruled out before a prescription is written. A resident being up late at night by itself does not justify the use of medications. This is particularly true of residents diagnosed with dementia or Alzheimer's disease. For these individuals, a phenomenon known as "sleep reversal" is not uncommon. This causes the individual to sleep sparingly at night and nap often during the day.

Once the medication order is written, it cannot be forgotten. The need for the medication to continue to be given must be regularly reassessed. In fact, the drug should not be given for longer than 10 days without an attempt to gradually reduce the dosage. There must also be documentation proving that the use of the drug has resulted in *maintenance of or improvement in the resident's functional status.* That means that if the drug is not measurably improving the problem or is causing other problems as well, it should be discontinued. A prime example of such a problem is what is known as "carryover," which results in the resident sleeping late into the day or being groggy, unsteady on his or her feet, or confused during the day.

In cases where the drug has been continued for more than 10 days, the rules call for at least three attempts to gradually reduce the dosage of the drug within six months. Each attempt must be documented in writing and if the medication is to be continued, the reasons for that decision also must be documented.

Finally, it must be understood that diminished sleep during the night is not uncommon among the elderly and is not necessarily a cause for concern or a justification for the use of medication. That decision should be based on whether it is causing negative impacts on the *person,* not whether the facility staff regard it as a problem. Commonly, the number of staff members during the night shift is significantly fewer than the day shift, so that the night shift staff may have difficulty rendering their care and making rounds sufficient to meet all the residents' needs while also having to supervise and ensure the safety of a resident who is moving about the facility. This can cause the facility to request the quick answer to the problem: drugs or restraints, especially if the resident is very confused, wanders, or is prone to falls.

The right answer to the problem is to improve the staffing levels on the night shift where that is necessary to improve supervision. The facility and the physician have the responsibility to address the problem in a manner that prevents the use of unnecessary drugs. Adequate staffing, door alarms, wanderer alert systems, quiet nighttime diversional activities, and medication review should all be considered before the use of a drug to manage sleep pattern problems.

Review of the medications already in use often reveals possible causes for sleep disturbances. Some common medications can cause insomnia, nightmares, or agitation among the elderly. Even the timing of administration of certain medications can contribute to the problem. For example,

Table 1. Anxiolytic and sedative drugs

Brand name	Generic name
Long-acting benzodiazepines	
Dalmane	Flurazepam
Librium	Chlordiazepoxide
Tranxene	Clorazepate
Valium	Diazepam
Klonopin	Clonazepam
Doral	Quazepam
Paxipam	Halazepam
Short-acting benzodiazepines	
Ativan	Lorazepam
Serax	Oxazepam
Xanax	Alprazolam
ProSom	Estazolam
Other common anxiolytic and sedative drugs	
Multiple brand names	Diphenhydramine
Atarax, Vistaril	Hydroxyzine
Multiple brand names	Chloral hydrate

giving a medication called a diuretic, commonly used to treat congestive heart failure, too late in the day can cause the resident to need to get up to the bathroom frequently during the night, because the drug increases urine output. Simply giving the medication earlier in the day can help prevent the problem. Informed residents or decision makers should ask questions about the other medications, dosages, and timing of administration when the facility wants to add a sleep-inducing drug to the care plan.

Problem behaviors include any *persistent* behavior that causes concern for the resident, family, decision maker, facility staff, other residents, and/or the physician. The response to those concerns should consider each of the following three perspectives:

1. The needs of the individual resident and family.

2. The impact the problem is having on other residents in the facility.

3. The viewpoint of the facility staff.

Table 2. Hypnotic drugs and barbiturates

Brand name	Generic name
Hypnotic drugs	
Restoril	Temazepam
Halcion	Triazolam
Ativan	Lorazepam
Serax	Oxazepam
Xanax	Alprazolam
ProSom	Estazolam
Benadryl	Diphenhydramine
Atarax, Vistaril	Hydroxyzine
Ambien	Zolpidem
Multiple brand names	Chloral hydrate
Doriden	Glutethimide
Noludar	Methprylon
Placidyl	Ethchlorvynol
Equanil, Miltown	Meprobamate
Multiple brand names	Paraldehyde
Barbiturates	
Amytal	Amobarbital
Butisol	Butabarbital
Nembutal	Pentobarbital
Seconal	Secobarbital
Multiple brand names	Phenobarbital
Tuinal	Amobarbital/secobarbital
Fiorinal	Barbiturates combined with other drugs

Table 3. Antipsychotic drugs

Brand name	Generic name
Thorazine	Chlorpromazine
Sparine	Promazine
Vesprin	Triflupromazine
Mellaril	Thioridazine
Serentil	Mesoridazine
Tindal	Acetophenazine
Trilafon	Perphenazine
Prolixin, Permitil	Fluphenazine
Stelazine	Trifluoperazine
Taractan	Chlorprothixene
Navane	Thiothixene
Haldol	Haloperidol
Moban	Molindone
Loxitane	Loxapine
Clozaril	Clozapine
Compazine	Prochlorperazine
Risperdal	Risperidone
Zyprexin	Olanzepine
Seroquel	Quetiapine

Tables 1–4 give the generic and brand names of some common drugs included in the various categories of psycho-active medications used in long-term care. The lists are drawn from the manual used by state survey agencies responsible for evaluating the quality of care and compliance with the regulations by long-term care facilities. Note that some drugs are considered to fall into more than one category.

■

POTENTIAL SIDE EFFECTS YOU SHOULD KNOW ABOUT

Any medication has the potential to cause side effects, the undesirable reactions that *may* result from the use of a

Table 4. Antidepressant drugs

Brand name	Generic name
Elavil	Amitryptyline
Asendin	Amoxapine
Norpramin, Pertofrane	Desipramine
Sinequan	Doxepin
Tofranil	Imipramine
Ludiomil	Maprotiline
Aventyl, Pamelor	Nortriptyline
Vivactil	Protriptyline
Surmontil	Trimipramine
Prozac	Fluoxetine
Zoloft	Sertraline
Desyrel	Trazodone
Anafranil	Clomipramine
Paxil	Paroxetine
Wellbutrin	Bupropion
Marplan	Isocarboxazid
Nardil	Phenelzine
Parnate	Tranylcypromine
Effexor	Venlafaxine
Serzone	Nefazodone
Luvox	Fluvoxamine

medication in addition to the desired therapeutic effects. Side effects can range from mild, temporary problems to severe, potentially permanent problems which can, if not addressed, lead to significant declines in the person's health and quality of life. One medication may have different side effects in different people, so the physician and the nursing staff of long-term care facilities need to know and observe for all symptoms of drug side effects. In this section, we focus on the known potential side effects of the category of psychoactive medications known as antipsychotic drugs. These drugs, when used in the right case and managed properly, can greatly enhance the quality of life for the person receiving them, but even if everything is done right, there are risks that consumers and decision makers need to know about.

In this section, we also look at what the facility must do to monitor the resident for the development of side effects. Since side effects may occur with the use of almost any medication, ask the facility to go over the known side effects with you (as a consumer or decision maker) before the initial use of the drug. When discussing the side effects, ask facility staff to explain the system they use for monitoring for side effects. OBRA requires that the facility have such a system; providing an explanation of it should pose no problem. Later in this chapter, we discuss some of the monitoring systems in use.

ORTHOSTATIC HYPOTENSION

This is a condition in which blood pressure drops abruptly when a person rises to stand from a seated or lying position. It can cause weakness, dizziness, and even fainting and falls. When a medication known to cause this side effect is started, or when the symptoms develop, the facility should be checking orthostatic blood pressures, which is done by checking the blood pressure when the person is lying down, then sitting up, and finally after rising to a standing position. Each blood pressure is noted, and if it drops significantly, a plan to deal with the problem is formulated.

The plan might include simple interventions like teaching the person to sit upright for a time before standing from a lying position. Also, teaching the individual to stand briefly by the chair or bed to make sure dizziness or weakness does not result or passes before walking away can help to prevent falls. Since this side effect is one that may pass with time, the medication may be continued, even if these symptoms do occur. For residents who are too confused or forgetful to be able to use the techniques just mentioned, the facility may need to consider trying an alternative medication or stopping the drug being given. Physical restraints may be considered under those circumstances, if used to *treat medical symptoms,* but if an alternative medication or approach to managing the behavior can be found, the restraint approach would not be necessary.

DROWSINESS

Drowsiness, or sedation, is a common side effect of a number of antipsychotic medications and in certain circumstances may even be considered beneficial. If drowsiness increases dependency on staff or has a detrimental effect on quality of life, alternatives will need to be tried. In some cases, drowsiness will pass with time or become less severe, but the facility should monitor the problem carefully and not let it continue too long.

When looking for alternatives, it is important to know that some medications that cause less drowsiness may present other side effects. For example, one drug may cause less sedation but involuntary muscle movement, called extrapyramidal symptoms. Thus one side effect may be exchanged for another that may actually be potentially more serious. Decision makers and family members must work closely with the physician and the facility staff when making choices about the use of antipsychotic medications.

Note: The facility is required to inform the resident or decision maker about the possible side effects of medications as a part of obtaining consent for their use.

ANTICHOLINERGIC EFFECTS

These effects, which interfere with the transmission of certain nerve impulses, result in symptoms that may seem relatively minor: thirst, constipation, dry skin, decreased perspiration, blurred vision, and urinary retention. More serious side effects can include confusion, visual or auditory hallucinations, depression, and psychosis. None of these side effects should be taken lightly if they diminish a resident's quality of life.

ABNORMAL INVOLUNTARY MUSCLE MOVEMENTS

There are several drug-induced syndromes involving muscle movement with different characteristics.

1. **Parkinsonism.** Symptoms include a fine, gradually spreading tremor, muscular weakness and rigidity, slow movements, drooling, expressionless or masklike face, slow speech, and blinking. As the condition worsens, symptoms may include poor balance and a slow, shuffling gait. This in turn may worsen to a forward-stooping posture accompanied by a gait that tends to start slowly and increase speed as the person's body leans more forward until control is lost and the person tends to fall forward. This effect is known as "festination." The arms may be held in a flexed position and the thumbs may turn in toward the palms, with thumb and fingers performing a "pill rolling" motion. Medications can be used to treat these symptoms, but if they are anticholinergic drugs, they will tend to have a compounding or *additive* effect on the side effects. In some cases, these symptoms fade over a period of months. Note that these drugs do not cause Parkinson's disease. The symptoms may mimic those caused by the disease, but while these symptoms may fade over time, Parkinson's disease is permanent and its symptoms do not fade.

2. **Akathisia.** Symptoms include constant restlessness, pacing, and anxiety or discomfort with the thought of sitting down. Sleep disturbance is common, because the person cannot stay at rest for any length of time. The individual may report the sensation of muscle quivering. These symptoms may require that the medication be withdrawn.

3. **Tardive Dyskinesia.** Symptoms include slow, rhythmic repetitive motions, such as involuntary tongue protrusion, chewing motions, blinking, tics, grimacing, lip smacking or movement, tongue tremors, twisting of the neck, finger or toe movements, writhing of the

trunk of the body, ankle flexing, and foot tapping. These symptoms, if allowed to become severe enough, will have a debilitating effect. This makes the person increasingly dependent on caregivers, negating the goal of OBRA, which is to advance the person to her or his highest level of function and independence. In addition, research has shown that many of these symptoms remain and may be permanent, even after the drug has been discontinued. The risk of these side effects developing becomes greater with age, indicating that the typical long-term care resident is particularly vulnerable. Research has also shown that up to 40 percent of the elderly people receiving antipsychotic drugs over a long period of time will exhibit tardive dyskinesia and that it is irreversible in over 50 percent of all cases. If the situation is allowed to continue, the effects can become so profound that they may affect the ability of the person to eat, speak, drink, and even breathe, making these side effects potentially life-threatening.

■
MANAGEMENT AND MONITORING OF PSYCHOACTIVE DRUGS

CONSUMER GUIDELINES

The following checklist can help you as a consumer or decision maker ensure that psychoactive drug therapy is necessary and managed appropriately:

1. Before resorting to medication to deal with problem behaviors has the facility done a thorough physical assessment for possible causes of the behavior?

2. Have environmental factors been ruled out as the cause of the behavior?

3. Has a psychological evaluation been completed?

4. If no diagnosis of mental illness exists, what conditions or symptoms are being treated?

5. Is the proposed drug indicated (appropriate) for the condition to be treated?

6. Is the dose ordered the smallest dose likely to have an effect?

7. Will dose reductions be tried and when?

8. When will the drug be withdrawn?

9. Will the drug be given on a regular schedule, as needed (designated "PRN"), or both?

10. If the facility can give it as needed, what are the specific reasons or behaviors that will justify the use of the drug? Are they specified in the orders?

11. Has the above information been thoroughly explained and have all your questions been answered as part of giving informed consent prior to the first dose being given? An exception to this requirement is when the facility received an order for immediate administration of the drug in an emergency situation. In that case, the facility must obtain consent for use within 24 hours of its use. The facility must then assess the cause of the behavior that led to the use of the drug and make every effort to treat the cause and reduce or eliminate the use of the drug.

12. If more than one psychoactive medication is in use, was consent obtained for each?

13. Is the proposed dose in line with the dose guidelines in the OBRA guidelines? If not, why? Ask the nursing staff to review the dosing guidelines with you.

14. If the psychoactive drugs were started during a hospital stay and are being continued in the nursing facility, has there been an assessment to determine whether the order is still necessary?

15. If the drug is to be discontinued, is it safe to have it stopped abruptly or must it be gradually tapered by decreasing the dose to prevent withdrawal symptoms?

16. Is the drug withdrawal a part of a plan to begin alternative treatment of the condition that led to its use in the first place and how will the new approach be monitored?

17. Is the drug being proposed actually going to treat the side effects of another drug already in use?

18. Is the desired effect of the proposed drug the same as any other drug already in use? If so, why would both drugs be used?

OBRA GUIDELINES

Because of the hazards associated with the use of psychoactive medications, OBRA has several specific requirements that must be adhered to:

1. The dose of the medication should be no greater than is absolutely necessary.

2. The drug should be discontinued as soon as it is no longer needed.

3. The reasons (indications) for its use should be appropriate.

4. Adequate monitoring should be in place.

5. The dose should be reduced or the drug discontinued if side effects develop that warrant these steps.

The manufacturers of medications recommend dosages for their products in the product literature. Generally, the manufacturer bases these recommendations on the patient's age and body weight and/or the form the medication is supplied in. The doctor must use judgment in taking into account other factors that affect the dose prescribed, such as the patient's physical condition and other medications already in use. Generally speaking, the greater the dose, the more quickly side effects will emerge and the more severe they will be. If the individual is ill or taking medications with an additive effect, the same will hold true.

Knowing when the use of a medication is no longer necessary fits hand-in-glove with knowing if it was necessary in the first place. Each decision depends on accurate assessment of the problem and its cause. To that extent, being able to identify in some quantitative form exactly how bad a person's behavioral symptoms are becomes the basis for meeting the requirements in OBRA. Once assessment systems are in place, the facility is then able to monitor for improvement or decline and guide the care planning process where the use of psychoactive medications is concerned.

BEHAVIORAL MONITORING

When a behavioral problem emerges, the facility may begin what is known as a **behavioral monitoring record.** This is a log for tracking specific behaviors that have been observed, the time of day or shift they occur, how often, and whether there any factors that seem to trigger the behavior. The log may provide enough information to allow the facility to identify a solution to the problem. If not, it can help to quantify the problem in terms of frequency and severity to help make decisions about whether medication is needed and, by ongoing monitoring, whether the medication is working. The log may also be useful in defining the proper time to give medications so that their peak effectiveness occurs when the behaviors have been most often observed. Such monitoring can also help gauge the success of drug withdrawal or substitute therapy.

In addition to monitoring the behaviors that may lead to the use of psychoactive medications, the facility must also monitor the side effects of the medications.

DRUG SIDE-EFFECT MONITORING

The Dyskinesia Identification System: Condensed User Scale (DISCUS) is a system for monitoring the onset of tardive dyskinesia. DISCUS screening allows properly trained facility staff to perform a physical assessment that looks at key symptoms of tardive dyskinesia and apply a numeric value to the symptoms observed. The scale ranges from 0 to 4, with 4 being used to indicate that the symptom was easily observed and severe. Properly done, ideally by the same clinician each time, the DISCUS screening provides a consistent basis for detection and measurement of psychoactive drug side effects.

Another tool, which is simply referred to as a dyskinesia monitoring record, uses the same rating scale and facilitates much the same assessment but also includes assessment of how much the abnormal movements incapacitate the resident, whether or not the person is aware of the abnormal movements, and the status of the resident's dental health (which helps prevent an ill-fitting upper plate from being mistaken for abnormal chewing motions). This tool also identifies how long the resident has been taking the psychoactive medications, the dose being given, the diagnosis, and whether the person is receiving medications to treat the side effects. Finally, this system uses a total score to facilitate overall comparisons to past measurements. This procedure is also referred to as the AIMS test, or Abnormal Involuntary Movement Scale.

OBRA does not select the system a facility uses or the frequency of monitoring. It only specifies that it must be "adequate." The fact is that hard-and-fast rules about type and frequency of monitoring may not work the same in all cases. Some authorities suggest that weekly blood pressure monitoring be done when orthostatic hypotension is a concern and that monthly assessments be done using DISCUS, AIMS, or some other system for medications known to place the resident at risk for abnormal involuntary muscle movements or tardive dyskinesia. If there are no obvious changes affecting the resident, it may be acceptable to perform the assessments as part of the quarterly review (see chapter 9), but it is unlikely that anything less frequent will be viewed as adequate.

No matter what system is in use, the facility must document baseline measurements so that changes can be accurately evaluated. All the assessment in the world will not help unless something results from it. If you are in the role of a decision maker, all of this must be clearly explained to you and you must be informed as to what, if anything, will be done in response to changes these monitoring activities show. Some of the questions you may wish to ask are the following:

1. If side effects are not occurring and behavioral monitoring shows improvement, when will dose reduction be tried?

2. If side effects are not occurring and behavioral monitoring shows no improvement, is it time to stop the medication and try another approach, starting with reassessment of the behaviors?

3. If side effects are occurring, how severe are they and are behaviors improving? Are the risks of worsening side effects worth the improvements that may have occurred?

4. If side effects are occurring and behaviors have not improved, when will the medication be discontinued and the situation reassessed?

The physician's advice in making decisions on this can be vital, so if you are in doubt about care planning issues discuss them with him or her and consult with the facility staff.

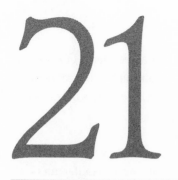

Don't Tie Me Down!

THE RIGHT TO BE FREE FROM THE
USE OF PHYSICAL RESTRAINTS

Even more widespread than the use of psychoactive medications and at least as controversial is the use of physical restraints in nursing homes. Devices and techniques that are considered physical restraints cover the range from the most obvious and restrictive methods such as "four-point" wrist and ankle restraints, to the subtle and *unauthorized* immobilization of a resident in bed by tucking the bed linen under the mattress so tightly that the resident cannot even change position without staff help.

By definition, a physical restraint is any "manual method or physical or mechanical device, material, or equipment attached to or adjacent to the resident's body that the individual cannot remove easily which restricts freedom of movement or normal access to one's body." This broad definition encompasses quite a range of devices and techniques. It also allows some devices and techniques to be considered restraints when used on one individual but not when used on another.

One of the key factors in determining whether a device constitutes a restraint is whether the resident can easily remove it himself or herself. In some cases, a device may be placed in use to keep a resident from being able to stand up and walk unassisted. This is one approach to the safety problems of a resident who has a very unsteady gait and is prone to falls. A facility may advocate the use of a lap belt type of restraint that has a buckle on the front and is secured to the back of a wheelchair or geriatric chair, behind the resident. Since the resident can easily reach the buckle, the facility may assert that the resident should be able to open the buckle independently and so is not really restrained. If the resident truly can open the buckle and remove the device unassisted, the device would constitute a "reminder" type of intervention and not be considered a restraint. The same device used on a resident who is unable to open the device because of profound dementia or severe arthritis of the hands would be considered a restraint.

A similar distinction must be drawn when side rails are used on a bed. Side rails that the resident cannot lower, if intended to keep the resident from getting out of bed unassisted, constitute a physical restraint. On the other hand, if they are used as a reminder to call for assistance, although the resident can lower them independently, they do not constitute a restraint. Also, if they are positioned so that residents can use them as "grab rails" for repositioning or to pull themselves up to a sitting position, side rails do not constitute a physical restraint. Unfortunately, there can be times when both the intent and the effect are unclear.

Despite being one of the lightning rod issues that led Congress to enact OBRA in the first place, and despite development of comprehensive guidelines in OBRA and massive amounts of work by clinicians, academics, and entrepreneurs, the use of physical restraints since OBRA became law has been reduced only incrementally nationwide. From 1991 (the first year for which comprehensive statistics are available) to 1997, the use of physical restraints declined only 5.9 percent nationwide, creeping down from 21.7 percent in 1991 to 15.8 percent (see figure 7). This statistic demonstrates that survey teams and regulations alone cannot reduce the use of physical restraints—an informed public is necessary. The following OBRA rules apply when physical restraints of any type are in use:

1. The facility must conduct a thorough assessment of the resident's condition and try alternatives to the use of a physical restraint before implementing any restraint.

2. The facility must define an approach using the least restrictive device or technique possible and for the least time possible. Whatever device is selected, it must be necessary to *treat the resident's symptoms.*

3. The facility must conduct ongoing assessment of the resident's condition and discontinue the device or move to a less restrictive device as soon as possible.

4. No restraint can be applied without written consent of the resident or her or his decision maker (except in defined emergency situations for limited periods of time).

5. No restraint can be applied without a physician's order. The type of restraint, times of application, where it may be applied, how long it may be applied, and under what circumstances it may be applied should be specified in the order or in the resident's care plan.

6. The use of the restraint must be reevaluated by the physician on rounds and by the facility quarterly.

7. The facility must document its assessments of the signs of adverse side effects of restraint use in the resident's medical records (more detail on side effects of restraint use later).

8. The restraint must be released every two hours for toileting, walking, and exercise. Most manufacturers recommend that the restraint should be checked every half hour for proper fit and application.

9. The resident's call light button must be kept in reach while the restraint is on.

10. The resident must be checked for incontinence, sources of discomfort, and skin breakdown.

11. The staff should offer water or other fluids between meals and assist the resident as needed to ensure the resident actually gets fluid intake.

12. The staff must ensure items the resident routinely uses are within reach when the restraint is on: personal items like combs, reading materials, and, of course, the remote control for the television.

13. The resident must be assured of opportunities to participate in diversional activities. If the restraint inhibits the ability to do that independently, then the staff must make the additional effort to assist the resident to any chosen activities.

To provide a better basis for you to understand this issue as a consumer or as a decision maker, we take a look at some of the common devices used as physical restraints.

■

TYPES OF DEVICES USED AS PHYSICAL RESTRAINTS

LAP BELT OR WAIST RESTRAINT

This is a padded beltlike device sometimes referred to as a "Posey," after the name of one of the major manufacturers

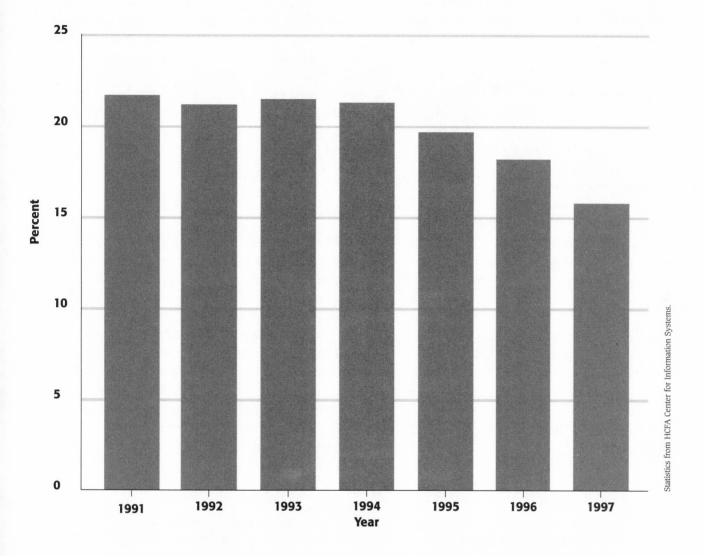

Statistics from HCFA Center for Information Systems.

Use of physical restraints decreased from 21.7 percent in 1991 to 15.8 percent in 1997. Consumers should view even this modest improvement cautiously since many facilities consider a resident to be "restraint-free" when a device that is not actually fastened to the resident is in use, such as a reclining chair, even though the resident in many instances cannot rise from the chair to walk or toilet independently.

of restraints.[1] The belt is fitted around the resident's waist so that it fits across the hips, not the abdomen. It should be placed in much the same position as an automobile seat belt. It is then threaded beneath and behind the wheelchair or geriatric chair seat, with the tie straps crossing and then fastened to the underframe of the chair. Some versions of the lap belt have a buckle on the front or a Velcro closure, enabling the resident who is physically or mentally capable to remove it. The fastening to the underframe must be done with quick-release slip knots or buckles designed to be released quickly so the device can quickly be removed in the event of an entanglement. The attachment points must be designed to avoid their slipping along the underframe, causing the device to become looser or tighter. The lap belt is *not* to be simply tied around the backrest of the chair and allowed to lie over the person's abdomen or chest. This can cause discomfort and is likely to constrict the person's ability to breathe, particularly if the person slides down in the chair.

This device must *not* be attached tightly around the waist but should not have excessive slack, either. This type of device has been implicated in serious injuries and fatalities when the resident has been able to slide forward and down in the chair, so that the belt compresses the chest, causing suffocation. The potential for injury exists even when the device is properly applied.

A variation of the waist restraint called a **groin restraint** or **pelvic restraint** is also available but infrequently used these days. This is a lap belt with a padded extension that drops down between the resident's legs, under the buttocks, and attaches to the back of the chair frame to prevent the resident from sliding forward. This device can be uncomfortable and lead to skin abrasion and breakdown problems, particularly when used on incontinent residents.

VEST OR JACKET RESTRAINT

This type of device fits much like a vest or jacket, as the name implies, but it has cloth or nylon straps that pass be- hind the resident and attach to the chair in much the same way as the lap belt. This device poses the same potential injury hazards as the lap belt. Some versions of this device are of a "wraparound" design, which becomes more snug if the resident slides forward in the chair, inhibiting the movement, but it can in the same way put more pressure in the skin contact areas. This type of device is sometimes incorrectly put on backwards, so that the neck opening impinges on the person's throat. If you observe this improper application, notify the nursing staff at once. Properly applied, the device should have a V-neck or scoop-neck appearance in front.

POSTURAL DEVICE

This device may resemble a vest or jacket restraint, or it may look more like a padded harness that is designed to fit around the chest. Typically, the device will have ties or buckles on straps that close behind the backrest of a wheelchair or geriatric chair. The device is intended to assist the resident maintain an upright posture by preventing leaning too far forward or side-to-side. Since the device generally will not be able to be removed by the resident independently, it must be considered and managed as a restraint. The ties and buckles must be of the quick-release variety and the device must be checked and released just as frequently as any form of restraint. Proper application and monitoring are essential to ensure resident comfort and safety.

A variation on the postural device is an **orthotic postural device** or **torso support.** It is designed to be secured to a chair with straps and may include an integral seat cushion. A support jacket with vertical plastic ribs in it wraps around the resident's trunk and closes in front with straps and buckles. The device is a good intervention for individuals who are unable to maintain normal body alignment while sitting. The device must be considered a restraint if the resident is unable to open it independently, even though the buckle closures are on the front in easy reach, or if it prevents movement the person could otherwise make.

---

1. Posey is a registered trademark of the Posey Co., Arcadia, California. Posey offers excellent training materials on the sale and appropriate use of physical restraining and safety devices. For more information, contact Posey Co. at 1-800-447-6739.

Each of these devices may be very helpful in some cases, but they are often unnecessary when the resident can be supported in a comfortable position with pillow bolsters on one or both sides of the body when the resident is sitting up. Simple, safer, and more comfortable interventions should be considered in solving body alignment problems.

ROLL BELT OR ROLLING BED RESTRAINT

This device is a wide, padded belt that starts with a tie or quick-release buckle on one end, and is designed to course around the person's waist, pass through a slot in the device, and continue on to a tie or buckle on its other end. Each end of the device attaches to the frame of the bed. The device is designed for use only while the resident is in bed and allows the resident to roll from side to side but not to get out of bed.

Proper application is critical to resident safety with all restraints, and any device that is applied to a person in a hospital bed should be applied to the portion of the bed frame that moves when the head of the bed is raised or lowered. If it is not, the device will tighten or loosen as the head of the bed is raised or lowered. This type of device may be used with only limited effectiveness in the case of very confused residents who are mobile and active. The use of any device may pose a greater hazard to the resident's safety than using a bed alarm (discussed later in this chapter) or no restraint at all and improved supervision.

Vest restraints have been used for residents in bed in some facilities, but they afford virtually no freedom to change position independently for the resident and may not be a safe choice, even for short periods of time. An exceptionally dangerous practice is to attempt to use a standard lap belt designed for use in a chair as a bed restraint by simply tying it across the resident to each side of the bed. It is not designed for this application, offers no security, and poses a high risk of strangulation to the resident.

WRIST AND ANKLE RESTRAINTS

A wrist restraint is a padded strap that buckles or ties around the wrist. It may be made of cloth or leather and have a buckle or Velcro closure. These devices are used in the nursing facility setting rarely, generally only when the resident's hands must be restrained to prevent the resident from pulling out an IV or feeding tube or in the case of extreme resident aggression. The use of this device is confined to the shortest possible time.

Ankle restraints are basically the same as wrist restraints; when used together with wrist restraints, they are referred to as **four-point restraints.** Such restraint in the nursing facility setting can be justified only in the most extreme circumstances and for the shortest period of time. The use of such devices tends to occur more often in the acute mental health care setting.

Limb restraints are among the most restrictive and disempowering devices that can be used in long-term care, so their use must be absolutely necessary, carefully monitored, and discontinued at the earliest opportunity.

WHEELCHAIR SAFETY BAR

This is a padded bar that is inserted and secured into position across the front of the wheelchair. The bar prevents the resident from leaving the wheelchair independently. It has the advantage of not being in such close contact with the resident's body as a lap belt or vest restraint, but it calls attention to the fact the resident is restrained by its prominent appearance and can pose safety hazards of its own, such as entanglement if the resident slides down beneath the bar, pinch-points at the points of attachment, and skin tears or bruising if the resident attempts to defeat the device.

GERIATRIC CHAIR

This variant of the wheelchair, usually called a geri-chair, is designed to be difficult for the person in it to propel. Unlike the wheelchair, which has large drive wheels designed to allow the user to move the chair, the geri-chair has only small wheels, which are not intended to function in propelling the chair. Most models have a footrest, which can be extended out to the front to provide a comfortable seating position. In the retracted position, the footrest may allow enough room for the person to propel the chair independently with his or her feet, if the feet can reach the floor. This is seldom the case, and the resident who cannot reach the floor or whose footrest is extended is completely immobile without help.

The geri-chair has a removable tabletop that can lock into position across the armrests of the chair in front of the resident. When this is done and the footrest is extended, the person in the geri-chair is very immobile and dependent—unable to move the chair or get up independently. Since the tabletop is generally difficult for even an alert resident to remove from inside the chair, when it is up and locked in place, the chair could in most cases be considered a restraint.

Properly used the geri-chair can provide the resident with a safe, comfortable seating position, offering better support than most wheelchairs. Newer variations on this type of chair offer contoured seat cushions, fine upholstery, and reclining seating positions. The device can improve the quality of life of residents who truly need this type of intervention. The device should not be used only to reduce the difficulty of supervision by acting as a restraint while contributing nothing to the resident's quality of life.

RECLINING CHAIRS

Reclining chairs have come into wide use in long-term care. These chairs offer very comfortable seating and are appropriate for the resident who can benefit from the reclining position. However, these chairs are not appropriate for all individuals and circumstances. Placing a resident in a reclined position from which he or she cannot rise alone must be considered as a restraint. The generally attractive appearance of these devices may lead to a tendency on the part of the staff to leave the resident, who looks comfortable, in the chair, possibly in the same position for extended periods of time. Thus the staff fails to get the resident up for toileting, walking, skin care, and perhaps even routine repositioning.

The rationale for the use of the reclining chair in some cases is that if residents are weak and relatively immobile, placing them in a recliner may make it all but impossible for them to attempt to get up on their own, even if a lap belt or vest restraint is not used. Thus the facility may tend

to count the resident as being "restraint-free." That would be true only to the extent that the resident does not have the belt or vest device on. Beyond that, though, the resident is still totally dependent on the staff for mobility, toileting, getting to food and fluids, skin care, and exercise. In using the recliner the facility has used the least restrictive type of device perhaps, but the rules about checking on the resident, offering fluids, mobility, and performing incontinent care, turning, and repositioning apply just as though a belt or vest was applied.

MITT RESTRAINTS

Mitt restraints are used to impede a resident's ability to grasp, pinch, and scratch, and may be padded in such a way that they act like boxing gloves to minimize the chance of harm if the resident strikes out. Typically, the palm side of the device is thickly padded from the wrist to fingertips and the entire hand lies behind the padded area. The backside may also be padded or may be made of a mesh type of material to help keep the hands cool. The device is secured to the hands with a wrist strap or band. It is important that these not be fastened too tightly to avoid cutting off blood flow to the hand. This type of device should be used as sparingly as possible since it tends to make the resident very dependent on the staff for most daily activities.

LAP BUDDIES

A lap buddy is an upholstered foam rubber block that fits across the lap of a resident seated in a geri-chair or wheelchair. It is held in place by extensions under the armrests of the chair. Once in place, it keeps the resident from being able to stand up independently. The advantage of the device is that it should provide some space between the device and the resident's body; however, a large resident's body may not fit without some contact with the device on the thighs or abdomen. Its use in these cases should be considered very carefully, since such contact can cause pressure on the skin and potential discomfort for the resident.

■
LESS RESTRICTIVE DEVICES
AND TECHNIQUES

If you are your own decision maker or the decision maker for a loved one, the foregoing information should help you understand devices used as restraints. There are some other interventions that are used to achieve some of the same objectives that these devices are intended to achieve.

These devices do not necessarily meet the criteria OBRA uses to define a restraint, but they may have much the same effect as a restraint where resident independence of action and mobility is concerned. Consequently, even though these devices may be touted as alternatives to restraint or capable of making the resident restraint-free, it is often more accurate to consider these devices to be less restrictive approaches to resident safety. All of the effects of the use of such devices must be taken into account when developing the care plan. If the device renders the resident just as immobile or dependent for exercise, walking, repositioning, toileting, getting to food and fluids, and mobility around the facility, then the facility needs to provide for those things just as frequently as if one of the restraints listed in the last section were in use.

WEDGE CUSHION

At first glance, a device called a wedge cushion does not appear to be an item that could in any way restrain an individual. It can be considered a least restrictive type of intervention for some residents when posture and safety are two objectives. A wedge cushion is a vinyl upholstered cushion in the shape of a wedge designed to be placed in the seat of a chair with the highest side of the wedge across the front edge of the seat of the chair. The thinnest edge of the cushion is placed along the base of the backrest of the chair. This arrangement helps prevent the resident from sliding forward in the chair and the firm cushion provides better support than the sway-bottomed seat of a typical wheelchair.

Even though the cushion does not attach to the resident in any way—it has no belts or straps for that purpose—it can prevent some residents from being able to rise to a stand-ing position without assistance. This can happen when residents are unable to get their weight over the elevated edge of the cushion, enabling them to stand up. If this is the case, the resident is just as effectively restrained from getting up independently as when a lap belt is in use. The resident is dependent on the staff for assistance to get up for exercise and toileting, and the resident who is unable to move the chair about independently is also dependent for mobility, food, fluids, and activities. Thus it is important to treat the resident as though he or she has a restraint on if the resident is unable to get up when the wedge cushion is in use: the staff should check the resident often and provide for fluids, toileting, walking, exercise, and repositioning the person.

One final note on wedge cushions: when used in a wheelchair, the height of the footrests should be adjusted to ensure that the feet are supported, not left hanging in the air. This will prevent pressure behind the resident's knees from reducing blood flow to the lower legs.

BED AND CHAIR ALARMS

These devices are intended to alert the facility staff when a resident is attempting to leave a chair or bed unassisted. Some operate with a pressure-sensitive pad placed under a bed mattress pad or on the seat of a chair, which triggers an alarm sound when the pressure is released as the person attempts to stand up. This particular type of triggering mechanism may go off when the resident changes position, causing a lot of false alarms. Not only does this contribute unnecessary noise to the facility's environment; it can also desensitize staff members to the alert signal. Another device uses a tether line attached to the person's clothing. This type can be defeated by the resident who manages to disconnect the tether.

The beauty of these devices lies in the fact that they open the possibility that residents can be without a restraint or any other device that would inhibit their ability to move at their will. The device calls for assistance for them, wherever they are in the facility when they wish to stand and walk. Such devices also can act as reminders to residents that they need assistance to walk, leading them to sit back down after the alert signal sounds. Though such devices may cost more than $100, it may be worth the facility's investment to use them when they are appropriate and can help keep a resident both safe and restraint-free.

WANDERER ALARMS AND DOOR ALARMS

These high-tech devices protect the resident who is prone to wander. The wanderer alarm system uses a tiny radio transmitter in a bracelet worn on ankle or wrist. The facility installs at each exit radio receivers that are connected or can transmit a signal to an alarm panel at the nurse's station. When the resident wearing the transmitter gets within a few feet of the receiver at the door, the system activates an alarm at the panel and may sound an alarm at the door location, alerting the staff that the resident is in a position to leave the building.

If the resident is able to remove the transmitter bracelet or if the transmitter fails, the system is defeated. In an effort to prevent this, the facility needs to check the transmitters and door receiver at least daily. The manufacturers of such devices make equipment for the purpose of checking the transmitters and receivers. If such a system is to be used for your loved one, ask how often the system is checked.

These systems, like the chair alarm, can send false signals (other electrical equipment such as floor buffers and vacuum cleaners may cause false alarms); moreover, the system must be maintained daily and the staff must be trained to use the system. Nevertheless, such systems are an excellent investment for a facility seeking to allow wandering residents maximum freedom to move about while ensuring a high degree of safety. Unfortunately, investment is part of the problem in encouraging the use of such systems— the cost can exceed $1,000 per door to set up. Both cost and complexity have kept wanderer alarm systems from being in wide use. Instead the cheaper and simpler door alarm system is in very common use and, while it is better than no security system, it is not without its problems.

The simple door alarm system sounds an alarm every time the exit door is opened. This is accomplished by a mechanical or magnetic switch. These systems are of very limited value because the alarm system can be switched off and the alarm sounds every time the door is open (assuming the system is turned on). The fact that the alarm sounds every time the door is opened leads to two weaknesses: the staff may tend to ignore the alarm and the system may tend to create so much noise that it is turned off most of the time. Residents eloping from the facility (leaving unaccompanied) is not an uncommon occurrence with these systems, so it is important to inquire about security procedures at the facility if you are the spouse or decision maker for an individual known to wander.

AMBULATORS

Ambulators, which came into use in the early 1990s, are growing in popularity. The device, which literally encloses the person using it, rather resembles a walker with a chair or stool built in. It has a frame made of metal tubing or white plastic pipe similar to the type used for plumbing, four wheels, and is designed to be used much the same way a walker is used, with the resident holding on to the frame and rolling the device along while walking. Residents can stand up inside the device to walk but sit down and rest in the seat of the device when they tire or feel unsteady. They also have the option of scooting the device along with their feet while seated.

The device affords a high degree of independent mobility and safety for residents who may have very little endurance or have an unsteady gait. The resident using the device tends to require less supervision than a resident who is restrained in a wheelchair or geri-chair. However, since the device is not designed to allow the resident to do everything independently, toileting, for example, the staff must still be alert to resident needs.

Though ambulators cannot offer an absolute guarantee against falls (no device can), they do offer an excellent alternative to the use of a restraint in a wheelchair for residents with gait problems, poor endurance, or cognitive impairments.

UNAUTHORIZED TYPES OF RESTRAINTS

As undesirable as the use of any physical restraint may be, the use of a properly designed device in the way the device was designed to be used at least gives the greatest likelihood of safe, effective use. When a restraint is patched together or a legitimate device is used improperly, the possibility of disaster is high.

There are techniques, some of which are rather subtle, that have been used in the past and no doubt are attempted today in some facilities, that consumers should be aware of. These practices are *never* ordered by a physician and are thus not to be used. Whenever they occur, these practices are unauthorized and they are dangerous to the resident. If you discover the use of any of these techniques and you are a family member, decision maker, or friend of a resident on whom the technique is being employed, notify the facility staff at once and insist that the situation be corrected immediately.

BED LINEN MUMMY WRAP

The practice of literally wrapping the resident in his or her bed top sheet and then covering the resident with the blanket, to obscure the restraint, is very dangerous. A variation of this is to tuck the top sheet under the mattress so tightly that the resident is virtually unable to change position or get up independently. Even when there is a legitimate order for the use of restraints, this technique is not allowed. These techniques pose a high degree of danger of entanglement and injury to the resident.

LAP ROBES OR SHAWLS

Many facilities provide lap robes or lap shawls to help keep the resident's legs warm and ensure privacy. Those are the only two approved purposes for the lap shawl. However, since most lap shawls have tie straps to help keep them from sliding off the resident's lap, there is the possibility of their misuse as a restraint as well. If the shawl has ties, they should be secured only around the resident's waist—

not tied to the chair itself. Tied to the chair, the shawl will act like a restraint and can pose a significant hazard to a resident when used this way. Even if a lap belt restraint is ordered for use when the resident is up in a chair, this technique is not acceptable.

TIE STRAP MISUSE

The tie straps of a legitimately ordered restraint device can be misused to immobilize a resident already restrained in a wheelchair. By threading the tie straps of a lap or vest restraint through the spokes of a wheelchair's wheels, the chair can be effectively locked in place. This technique is never acceptable and is generally used in an attempt to make supervision of very confused residents more convenient for the staff member who uses it. Since it may cause the restraint to get looser or tighter as the resident struggles to mobilize the wheelchair, this technique is very dangerous. It is contrary to the instructions for proper use of any lap or vest restraint.

TETHERING A CHAIR

Another unauthorized technique that may be attempted to minimize the mobility of a resident in a wheelchair is to tether the chair to some fixed object: a bed, handrail, or the like. This may be done using the tie strap of a legitimately ordered restraint device or by using another form of tie to make the attachment. This is not an acceptable technique and can pose dangers to the resident, particularly if the resident must be mobilized quickly in an emergency situation or if the ties of the restraint are misapplied to accomplish it. As with the previous technique, its only purpose is staff convenience, and it is prohibited on that basis under the OBRA reforms.

THE RIGHT DEVICE, BUT THE WRONG WAY

There are times when legitimate techniques may be used in inappropriate circumstances. An approved device or technique may be used when it is not necessary, in a way that is not intended by the manufacturer, or when it is not ordered by a physician, for instance. Note the following possible mistakes.

SETTING WHEEL LOCKS

Setting the wheel locks of a wheelchair, an essential technique in ensuring resident safety, is taught in all nursing assistant training programs. It is essential to do when it is necessary for the wheelchair to remain in one place for any reason, such as when the resident is being transferred into or out of it. The chair also must stay in place at the curbside while a resident is waiting to board a transfer van; though the resident must not be left unsupervised in such a circumstance, if someone is not actually in control of the resident's chair, the wheels must be locked to prevent unexpected movement.

Beyond these circumstances, however, the wheel locks should generally be left unlocked to allow the resident to mobilize the wheelchair if the resident is unable to lock and unlock the wheels independently. For a resident who is unable to unlock the wheels due to a cognitive impairment, weakness, or arthritic pain, setting the wheel locks can amount to restraining the resident in one place. If it is done for no reason other than staff convenience, it is prohibited by the regulations.

MISUSING LAP BELT RESTRAINTS

Use of a lap belt or any other type of restraint while the resident is using a toilet, bedside commode, or shower chair is extremely dangerous. Most facilities have a policy prohibiting this practice and all should. Applying any restraint under these circumstances is not consistent with the application recommendations of any manufacturer. A confused, unsteady resident must not be left unattended while toileting and certainly must not be left restrained in such a circumstance.

If the resident loses balance or struggles against the restraint, he or she is likely to fall; the restraint offers no safeguard against a fall and will probably inflict more injury than the fall itself. Bedside commodes and shower chairs are so light that if a restraint is attached to them, they will only be pulled over on top of the resident in the event of a fall.

■
RULES GOVERNING THE USE OF RESTRAINTS

OBRA's rules governing the use of physical restraints are as follows:

> *The resident has the right to be free from any chemical or physical restraints imposed for the purposes of discipline or convenience, and not required to treat the resident's medical symptoms. The intent of this requirement is for each person to reach his/her highest practicable well-being in an environment that prohibits the use of restraints for discipline or convenience and limits restraint use to circumstances in which the resident has medical symptoms that warrant the use of restraints.*
>
> *[42 CFR Sec. 483.13(a)]*

The intent of the OBRA requirements affecting the use of physical and chemical restraints is clear and unequivocal. The use of restraints for convenience of the facility or its staff and the use of restraints for disciplinary purposes are both *flatly prohibited.*

There are no exceptions to the prohibitions on the inappropriate use of restraints and none should be inferred. If a facility employs the use of physical restraints or psychoactive drugs which act as chemical restraints to offset understaffed units, the facility is allowing such uses for its own convenience. The medical necessity for the use of any form of restraint must be clear before any restraint is used and the facility is obligated to ensure that no properly ordered restraint is improperly applied or inadequately monitored and that no unauthorized form of restraint is ever used.

The tough part of the staffing issue is that the requirements for staffing levels in the facility may be met by the facility on paper yet still be inadequate to fully meet the needs of all the residents in the facility's care and create difficulty for the staff to adequately supervise residents. This leads residents who are forgetful or cognitively impaired and who are prone to falls to be at risk for being restrained based on the argument that "it's for their own safety," even though the real issue is adequate supervision.

Although the rules require that the facility have adequate staff to meet the care needs of the residents, proving that a facility is failing to do so could require a daunting amount of documentation. Most facilities do make an ongoing effort to hire and retain sufficient trained staff. The simple fact is that in many localities there are not enough qualified people available and the wages paid for nursing assistants are simply too low to compete with many other forms of employment. Chronic short staffing is one of the most common problems in long-term care facilities, and it can play a role in many quality-of-care issues from skin breakdown and abuse to inappropriate use of restraints.

All things considered, the mission to keep people living in long-term care facilities free from restraints must be carried out on a case-by-case basis. One of the primary goals of this book is to inform residents, family members, and decision makers how to go about doing that.

■

NO RESTRAINT SHOULD BE APPLIED UNTIL . . .

The reasons for applying any restraint must be clear and documented in writing. Therefore, no physical or chemical restraint should ever be applied to any resident until a thorough assessment of all the factors that may be the cause of problems or behaviors necessitating the restraint has been completed, alternatives have been tried and have failed, informed consent has been obtained, and the physician has given appropriate orders. (Emergency use of a restraint is excepted from the requirement these steps occur before the restraint is applied.) Even if all of these steps

have been completed, the use of the restraint should be for the most limited circumstances possible and for the shortest time period possible.

Throughout this process the resident and/or decision maker must be kept informed of the issues, the interventions being attempted, the alternatives, the risks and benefits, and whether progress is being made. The process for ongoing assessment of the need for restraints is outlined in OBRA:

1. What are the symptoms that led to the consideration of the use of restraints?

2. Are the symptoms caused by failure to

   ■ Meet individual needs?

   ■ Use aggressive rehabilitative/restorative care?

   ■ Provide meaningful activities?

   ■ Manipulate the resident's environment, including seating?

3. Can the causes of the symptoms be removed?

4. If the causes cannot be removed, have alternatives to restraints been tried?

5. If alternatives have been tried and have failed, is the least restrictive method used for the shortest period of time?

6. Does the facility monitor and adjust care to avoid negative outcomes while continuing to seek less restrictive alternatives?

7. Did the resident or decision maker make an informed choice, with full understanding of the risks, benefits, and alternatives?

8. Does the facility use the Resident Assessment Protocol (see chapter 9) on physical restraints to evaluate the appropriateness of restraint use?

9. Has the facility reevaluated the need for a restraint, made efforts to eliminate its use, and maintained the resident's strength and mobility?

Informed consent must be obtained in writing from the resident or resident's decision maker before the restraint is used. If a restraint is applied in an emergency situation, the facility must obtain orders and written consent within 24 hours. (This time is required to be no more than 12 hours in some states.) "Informed consent" means the decision maker must be supplied information about the risks, benefits, and side effects of the use of the proposed form of restraint.

Even after consent is given, the assessment process must continue. The fact that a person is in a restraint cannot be forgotten by the facility. The need for the restraint and assurance that the resident is not declining as the result of restraint use must be reassessed on an ongoing basis. *It is possible to withdraw consent for the use of a restraint.* This is an important decision and like all health care treatment decisions should be taken only after careful consideration of the potential consequences. The decision to withdraw consent and terminate the use of a restraint should be taken only after weighing the facts and conferring with facility staff and the attending physician. Withdrawal of a restraint, just like the process of implementing it in the first place, should be done with a team planning process, based on sound reasons.

What types of things should be looked at as a part of the assessment process? The Resident Assessment Protocol (RAP), which is part of the Resident Assessment Instrument, provides an excellent framework for the assessment process that asks the following questions:

1. Why is the restraint being proposed?

2. What type of restraint is being proposed for use?

3. During what times of day would it be applied?

4. Where will it be in use: in the resident's room, at all times when up in a chair and/or in bed?

5. How long may the restraint be applied each day?

6. Is the restraint to be applied under certain circumstances only? The circumstances where restraint use is allowed must be clearly identified in the physician's order.

7. Were there behaviors that caused the use of a restraint to be proposed? Have the causes for the behavior been thoroughly assessed? If a restraint has been in use, have the behaviors that caused the restraint to be ordered continued or abated? The protocol calls for the seven days previous to the date of assessment to be considered for the purposes of making this determination.

8. Is the risk of falls the main reason for proposing the use of the restraint? The RAP points out that the use of restraints has not been shown to safeguard residents from injury, but that fall prevention is "one of the most common reasons given by facilities for restraining residents." Careful assessment of the resident's fall history may reveal reasons amenable to treatment without restraints. For example, the use of psychoactive medications or antihypertensives may cause dizziness and thus contribute to falls or unsteady gait, but steps to minimize or eliminate these side effects could eliminate the suggestion of applying a restraint.

9. Is a restraint being proposed concomitant to certain treatments that are under way? If the resident attempts to dislodge an indwelling urinary catheter, a feeding tube, an IV line, or a surgical dressing, the use of restraint may be suggested. It is always necessary to consider whether such treatments are necessary and consistent with the resident's wishes (advance directive) and whether alternatives to the treatment have been considered. Temporary use of restraints for the purpose of administering necessary treatment is allowed, provided such treatment is consistent with the resident's advance directive and, if need be, is approved by the resident's decision maker.

10. Is the proposed restraint use intended to enable the resident to be more self-sufficient? This could be the case if the use of the device is to provide body support, such as a postural device. Proposed benefits must be

demonstrated and documented to be sure that they will, in fact, occur if the restraint is used.

11. If a restraint is already in use, what has been the response of the resident to the restraint? If the restraint causes anger or agitation and the resident continuously fights the device and caregivers, there is a chance the restraint may cause more harm than good. The resident may also respond to the restraint by passivity, withdrawal, signs of depression, or giving up. Responses at each extreme need to be assessed very carefully.

12. Have alternatives to the use of restraint been attempted and if so, is the device being proposed the *least restrictive* type available?

DANGERS AND IMPACTS OF RESTRAINT USE

Use of physical restraints can have physical and emotional effects on a person. OBRA requires that those potential negative effects be explained to the resident and/or decision maker as part of the informed consent process.

No discussion of the use of restraints can ignore the fact that fatal injuries have been associated with the use of physical restraints. Fatalities have resulted when residents become entangled in restraints or fall from bed or chair, causing the device to strangle or suffocate the resident. Restraints have contributed to fatalities less directly by causing falls that resulted in serious injuries and death from complications of those injuries. This is particularly noteworthy because the number of residents who can walk independently is declining (see figure 8).

The incidence of deaths and injuries has been significant enough to prompt the U.S. Food and Drug Administration (FDA) to issue warning bulletins to health professionals on those hazards in 1991. In 1995, the FDA also introduced restraint warning label requirements. The labeling is supposed to include warnings about the hazards associated with the use of restraints and information about the use of the device, such as the fact that restrictive devices can-

not be used without a physician's order. The possibility of injury exists even if the device is applied properly and all precautions are taken to prevent it.

BED SIDE RAILS POSE HAZARDS

Bed side rails have been implicated in a number of serious injuries and deaths. There are some ways to help reduce the possibility of such mishaps from occurring:

1. If a restrictive device is to be used while the person is in bed, full-length, one-piece side rails have been recommended. Further, they should be completely padded or covered to prevent the resident from going through the rails.

2. If a restrictive device is not in use, and the rails may be useful to assist the resident with independent bed mobility, partial-length rails (extending only about half the length of the bed) are recommended.

3. Use of partial-length rails in the raised position at both the head and foot portion of the bed has been discouraged as the result of injuries to people who become entrapped between the rail sets as they try to get out of bed by going between the two.

The 1995 *FDA Safety Bulletin* stated that in just over five years, the FDA had received 102 reports of "head or body entrapment incidents" involving bed side rails. It stated that "the 68 deaths, 22 injuries and 12 entrapments without injury occurred in hospitals, long-term care facilities and private homes." The report stated that all of the entrapments occurred in one of the following ways:

1. Through the bars of an individual side rail.

2. Through the space between split side rails.

3. Between the side rail and the mattress.

4. Between the headboard or footboard, side rail, and mattress.

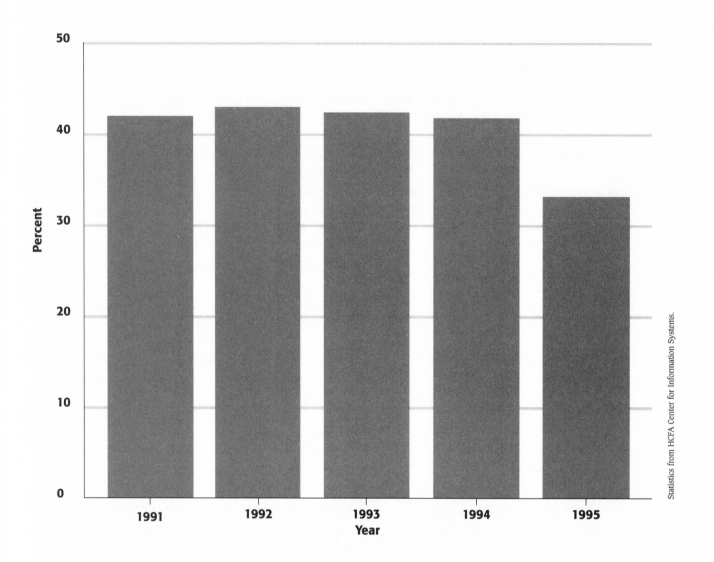

The number of nursing facility residents able to walk independently is declining. In 1991, some 42 percent of the nation's nursing home residents could get up and walk independently. By 1995, that number had fallen to just 33.2 percent. This may be a reflection of the trend toward ever higher degrees of acuity of condition among people admitted to nursing homes.

Statistics from HCFA Center for Information Systems.

Some long-term care facilities may use old hospital beds they can obtain more economically than new beds. Such beds may have had the original side rails removed. Replacement side rails may not fit the bed frame properly, resulting in loose fit, large gaps, or improper raising, lowering, or locking into position. Such side rails are unacceptable; if you notice such problems, report the problem to the facility administration.

THE SAFE MEDICAL DEVICES ACT

The Safe Medical Devices Act of 1990 (SMDA) requires hospitals, long-term care facilities, and other users of medical equipment to report injuries associated with the use of a medical device (restraints, wheelchairs, beds and side rails, etc.). The FDA has set up a hot line for health care providers to call in order to make such reports, but the FDA is interested in hearing from consumers as well. If you are aware of an injury or death associated with the use of a medical device, you can report it to MedWatch, the FDA's voluntary reporting program, at 1-(800) FDA-1088, or you can write to Medical Product Reporting Program, MedWatch, HF-2, Food and Drug Administration, 5600 Fishers Lane, Rockville, MD 20857.

This section has included more information on the possibility of death or injury resulting from the use of restraints and bed side rails than one would be likely to be given as part of most informed consent procedures in health care facilities. The case cannot be overstated because the possibility of such injuries is very real and should be a part of the "risk/benefit" analysis that must precede the use of restraints. Do not fear the use of restraints but be sure that all alternatives have been considered before a restraint is employed. There can be clear benefits derived from the appropriate use of the right type of restraint at the right time for the right reasons. The goal here is to help consumers understand the issue well enough to better judge when the risks are outweighed by the benefits and to understand the motivations a facility may have in recommending the use of physical restraints over other interventions.

■
SIDE EFFECTS OF THE USE OF PHYSICAL RESTRAINTS

There are other less ominous but certainly very important impacts on a person in restraints that need to be included in considering their use. Some of these impacts can be observed almost immediately. Others will develop over time, requiring skilled observation to note their earliest signs of onset.

The side effects described in this section will not necessarily occur in every case where a physical restraint is used and certainly not all of them should be expected to occur in any case, but it is not uncommon to have more than one of them occur, and the longer a restraint is in use, the greater the likelihood that more of them will occur. Precautions that can be taken to prevent these side effects from taking their toll on the restrained individual are discussed with each problem listed. If the side effects are still noted, consumers should discuss the problem with the facility. Reasonable consumers may ask to see the documentation of the facility's interventions to prevent these side effects from occurring.

MUSCLE WEAKNESS

The less muscles are used, the weaker and smaller they become. The rules in OBRA require that a restraint be checked and released at least every two hours for walking, exercise, and toileting. The presence of a physical or restorative therapy program of some type does not alter these requirements. The order for the use of restraints should specify these checking and release parameters; if assisted ambulation (walking) is necessary, the distance the resident should walk should also be specified. These guidelines are *minimums* set by OBRA. If the resident's condition indicates more frequent walking and exercise are needed to prevent muscle wasting and weakness from occurring, then the facility must comply. Good ways to do this are through a restorative nursing or therapy program, which augments the routine daily nursing care in this regard.

JOINT IMMOBILITY

Anyone who has exited an automobile after a long period of driving can probably relate to this problem—joints feel stiff and sore and may not want to move as they normally would. Being held in a seated or lying position by a restraint for extended periods of time has the same effect. If this occurs day after day, the problem can become more serious than the temporary stiffness of a long car trip.

The less often a skeletal joint is moved, the greater the likelihood of it becoming stiff, sore, and immobile. Maintaining flexibility is dependent upon frequent use. The same orders that prevent muscle weakness will help preserve joint mobility, but it is necessary for the facility nursing staff to help preserve joint mobility by ensuring that some simple **range of motion (ROM)** exercises are done at least twice a day to keep joints mobile. These exercises should be done routinely for any resident who has or is at risk for impaired mobility due to the use of restraints. A doctor's order is not necessary for the facility to provide ROM exercises; indeed, it is an expectation in the delivery of day-to-day care.

Range of motion exercises are of particular importance for residents with restraints in frequent use and/or with medical conditions, such as stroke-induced paralysis, that leave the resident unable to move joints voluntarily. In such cases, the staff provides all the movement to the affected joints for the resident: this is called **passive range of motion (PROM).** When the resident is able to perform the exercises independently or with minimal staff assistance, it is called **active range of motion (AROM).**

CONTRACTURES

A contracture is the disfigurement of a joint that has been left immobile for long periods of time, causing the muscles that move the joint to shorten, pulling the joint into a closed, contracted position. Individuals suffering from paralysis to a limb are most at risk for development of contractures, but very weak, debilitated individuals are also at risk, especially if they are further immobilized by the use of restraints. Regular, well-performed range of motion exercises can prevent contractures in virtually all cases. When restraints are in use, it is fair to ask the facility how often

ROM is performed if you are the decision maker for an individual who would benefit from such care. Range of motion exercises are often performed during residents' morning care, as part of their bathing and dressing. It should be performed again in the evening and more often during the day for those who are restrained or have conditions such as paralysis that place them at high risk. If you are a decision maker for a resident at risk and you believe you see evidence of the development of contractures, discuss it with the facility and the physician. A specific care plan can be developed to prevent contractures. Once that is done, keep an eye on the problem to ensure the care plan is being followed. Contractures are much easier to prevent than to correct.

INCONTINENCE

Incontinence is the loss of control over bowel or bladder. There are physical reasons this can happen, but the use of restraints can impose it on a resident who may not otherwise be incontinent. Even though OBRA calls for regular restraint release for toileting, the human body's schedule may not conform to the restraint release schedule. This problem is aggravated if the facility is too short-staffed to uphold the required release schedule. If the resident is aware of the need for toileting and is able to communicate that need, short-staffing or any other cause for a delay in assistance to the bathroom can cause tremendous frustration, discomfort, and embarrassment for the resident who is forced to wait for assistance and is incontinent before that assistance is available. There are times when even the best trained, best intentioned nursing staff can have difficulty being available at the moment the restrained resident needs to use the bathroom.

The task is even more difficult because among the elderly, physiological changes in the body can cause the bladder to have less capacity, leading to a more frequent urge to void and allowing the person less time to void before an episode of incontinency occurs. This frustrates staff members who do not understand the changes, because they may feel that "I *just helped* that resident to the bathroom—they can't need to go again." The most difficult situation exists when a resident is aware but unable to communicate the need for toileting due to other impairments.

Adhering to the restraint release schedule requirements in OBRA or releasing more often, if the need exists, is the closest thing to a solution to this problem where individuals in restraints are concerned. Keeping residents restraint-free and independent with walking and toilet use to the greatest extent possible is the best answer of all.

SKIN BREAKDOWN

Skin breakdown (decubitus ulcers) is the result of three forces combining, each of which can be countered or prevented altogether:

1. Pressure on the skin.

2. Moisture on the skin.

3. Shearing forces on the skin.

Pressure on the skin is unavoidable—whether a person is lying down or seated, pressure will be exerted on the skin at the area bearing the person's weight (see figure 9). Normally, this poses no problem because body fat and muscle act as cushioning, the skin is normally dry, and the person can change position at will to relieve the pressure.

These factors may all change for an elderly or disabled individual in a long-term care facility. Frequently residents will experience weight loss due to loss of both body fat and muscle mass. The loss of muscle mass and fat layer can cause bony prominences to have far less padding between them and the skin. Pressure then is more concentrated on the skin as well as on the tiny blood vessels called capillaries, which carry blood and oxygen to the cells of the skin. When this goes on long enough, the tissue starves for blood flow, causing it to weaken.

This problem is compounded by incontinence. As described in the preceding section, incontinence causes the skin of groin, buttocks, and thighs to frequently be moist, and residents may not be able to easily and frequently change position due to the use of a physical restraint. The skin weakens if moisture from urine or stool remains in contact with it for long periods of time. This can lead to maceration, or softening of the skin. Shearing forces resulting from the person's weight sliding across bed sheets or across the cushion of the seat of a wheelchair as well as repositioning and transfers from bed or chair can cause this softened, weakened skin to abrade or break open.

Prevention of skin breakdown is a priority of long-term care facility staff, and it is vital to the well-being of the resident. Unfortunately, the use of restraints can increase the likelihood of skin breakdown. Skin breakdown that may be related to the use of restraints occurs frequently over the tailbone, near the top of the crease of the buttocks, at the back of the pelvis, on the buttocks themselves where the buttocks meet the thighs (in an area known as the gluteal fold), between the legs, in the groin, or to the scrotum. Other areas where breakdown may occur include the spine, heels or sides of the feet, elbows, shoulderblades, even the back of the head and ears. Sites in this latter group are most likely to be affected when the person is partially or totally bedbound.

Severity of skin breakdown is reported in four stages (usually written in Roman numerals):

I. Skin area is reddened but not broken. The redness is persistent and may take 20 minutes or more to resolve. This is a warning to the staff that the reddened area may possibly break down if preventive measures are not taken.

II. A shallow break in the skin involving the outermost layer of the skin, called the epidermis and the dermis. The stage II ulcer may look like an abrasion, scrape, or blister.

III. This is a break in the skin that goes through the skin and into the fatty layers, called the subcutaneous tissue. This is of particular concern for two reasons: it may indicate a serious lack of attention to the resident's care needs for skin care and repositioning and, since it breaches the skin completely, it makes the resident very susceptible to infection through the wound.

IV. A stage IV ulcer is a very serious wound that penetrates through the skin, subcutaneous tissue, and through the muscle, and it may even reach the bone below.

FIGURE 9: PRESSURE SORES AND BEDFAST STATUS, 1991–1995

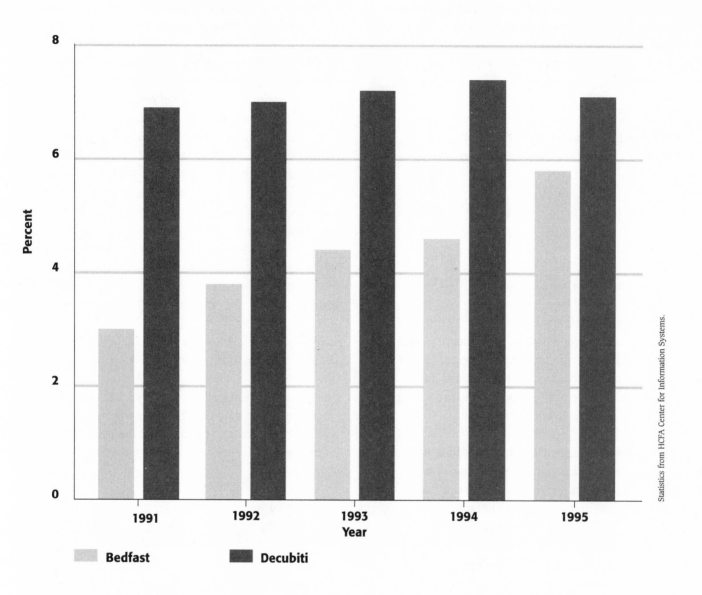

Statistics from HCFA Center for Information Systems.

Bedfast **Decubiti**

Despite myriad specialized products designed to prevent pressure sores (decubitus ulcers), progress in this area has been nil. The prevalence of pressure sores has increased from 6.9 percent in 1991 to 7.1 percent in 1995. This increase might have been worse, though, because the number of bedfast (spending all or most of their time in bed) residents increased even more: from 3 percent in 1991 to 5.8 percent in 1995. These residents are at greatest risk for pressure sores.

When skin breakdown is noted, the care plan must be reviewed; steps to deal with it and steps to prevent it in the future should be added. Decision makers should be informed that the problem has been noted and should be informed about what is being done to deal with the problem.

Prevention of skin breakdown is a priority, particularly for residents who are restrained. Some things that can be done to prevent breakdown include:

1. Adherence to the restraint check and release schedule.

2. Checking for incontinency frequently and providing immediate skin care if it has occurred. Keeping the skin clean and dry and keeping clothing and undergarments clean and dry. Barrier creams and lotions can help protect skin as well.

3. Use of pressure relief or pressure-reducing devices such as a gel cushion in the person's chair, convoluted foam rubber mattress overlays, air mattresses, water mattresses, or alternating pressure mattresses on the bed.

4. Frequent turning and repositioning for residents unable to do it themselves. Frequent exercise and time walking for those who are able to do that with or without assistance. Use of proper technique during transfers, turning, and repositioning is also of great importance. Placing a "lifter" in the chair or bed, underneath the resident, can make turning and repositioning easier for the staff and greatly reduce shearing forces on the skin. A lifter is a blanket, pad, or sheet positioned under the resident's body, which is grasped by the staff when lifting the resident, thus preventing sliding along the surface of the chair seat or bed linen.

5. Eliminate or reduce the use of physical restraints as soon as possible.

The importance of proper skin care in the long-term care facility setting is summed up in the expectations that OBRA has in regard to skin breakdown: persons admitted with no skin breakdown problems are expected to remain free of skin breakdown problems while in the facility unless their clinical condition makes skin breakdown unavoidable. If skin breakdown is occurring and there is no clinical condition that would tend to make such breakdown unavoidable, you as a resident and/or decision maker need to discuss this concern with the facility staff, find out why it is happening, and ensure that steps are taken to deal with it.

CONSTIPATION

The human bowel works best with the assistance of gravity and the stimulation of the body in motion: walking, turning, standing, and sitting. When the amount of activity decreases, the activity of the bowel, called motility, may also decrease. The bowel's rhythmic movement, called peristalsis, may slow down, causing fecal matter in the bowel to move more slowly through the digestive tract, lose moisture back into the walls of the intestines, and become harder and dryer. If constipation goes unremedied long enough, it can lead to severe constipation, called an impaction.

As with other complications of restraint use, prevention is relatively simple: the facility must ensure the restraints are released at least as often as required to provide for walking and toileting, provide plenty of fluids, adequate fiber in the diet, and, best of all, avoid, reduce, or eliminate use of restraints.

RENAL CALCULI

The urinary system depends on gravity to drain urine from the kidneys to the bladder. This is also augmented by body movement as with the digestive tract, but the urinary system does not have the muscular activity that the digestive tract has with peristalsis to help keep things moving. Consequently, long periods of inactivity may cause inefficient urine drainage from the kidneys, leaving the stagnant urine in the urinary system. This can cause minerals to coalesce into crystals that can grow into painful kidney stones, or renal calculi. This process is hastened if the resident's fluid intake is poor and the resident is dehydrated. Calculi development is a silent process until one reaches the size where it is too large to leave the kidney or it is large enough to become lodged in the ureter, which is the tube that drains urine from the kidney to the bladder.

Prevention of such stones can be accomplished by ensuring plenty of fluids are consumed by the resident and by restricting use of restraints to ensure adequate toileting and physical activities are provided.

CIRCULATORY IMPAIRMENT

This potentially serious problem can be the direct result of a restraint being applied too tightly or the resident struggling against the restraint or changing position. This condition should never be allowed to continue long enough to cause injury, but if it were not discovered, tissue damage, particularly to nerves, could result. Circulatory impairment can also be caused by the restrained individual being left in the same position too long. Signs of the problem include cold, discolored feet or hands or edema (swelling) in the extremities. The resident complaining of pain, numbness, or loss of sensation is a sign of the problem. These are the signs and symptoms that the facility staff is responsible for observing for when they check the restraint for proper fit and application.

WEIGHT LOSS

Weight loss has been associated with the use of physical restraints because of the loss of protein and muscle mass as the result of prolonged inactivity. Just as weightlifters are able to "bulk up," or increase muscle mass, by prolonged use of the muscles, the opposite effect can occur when muscles are not used: they *lose* bulk and mass. This process is called **atrophy.** Other factors associated with the use of restraints that can contribute to weight loss include depression, causing poor intake; constipation, which can also cause poor appetite; and the use of medications for each of these problems, which may cause loss of appetite and poor intake.

AGGRESSION

Frustration and anger arising from the use of restraints can cause the resident to struggle against the device, caregivers, and other residents. It takes no clinical training to understand that the idea of being held down in any way goes against a person's instinctive desire to be free to move around at will. Ironically, when the best solution is to find

less restrictive means or alternatives to the use of restraint, there may be a tendency to impose even more restrictive measures or add the use of psychoactive drugs. Such a combination must be used only after the search for acceptable alternatives has failed. When both are used, the resident's quality of life must be assessed carefully and the search for the least restrictive means must be considered an ongoing priority for the facility.

ABRASIONS, BRUISES, AND SKIN TEARS

These injuries can be the direct result of the device in contact with the body. Even well-padded and properly applied devices can cause injuries under the right circumstances. The more agitated or combative the restraint causes the person to be, the greater the likelihood that these types of injuries will occur.

This list does not cover all the adverse side effects that can occur as the result of the use of physical restraints. Consumers and decision makers in long-term care need to be aware that these and other side effects must be considered as part of the process of care planning when physical restraints are used. The number of possible side effects should lend weight to the argument in favor of trying every possible alternative *before* resorting to the use of restraints.

■
THE SEARCH FOR ALTERNATIVES TO THE USE OF PHYSICAL RESTRAINTS

The effort to avoid the use of physical restraints begins with assessment. The first and best step to deal with problems or behaviors that lead to the consideration of the use of physical restraint is to attempt to identify the cause of the problem and correct it—instead of resorting too quickly to restraints, which, as we have seen, can cause numerous problems of their own.

The most common reason for considering restraints is to prevent falls. This is often a first consideration if it is related to one of the causes for admission to the facility, such as series of falls at home resulting in a hip, femur, or other fracture. The cause for falls must be thoroughly assessed to determine if steps short of the use of a restraint can be taken to eliminate or minimize the possibility of falls.

Often, individuals with a history of falls have or had problems with dizziness or an unsteady gait in the past. It is important for the facility to assess *for itself* whether such problems still exist and not to continue to use a restraint merely because such a device was in use at another nursing home or in the hospital. The use of physical restraints in hospitals, by the way, is *not* regulated under OBRA, so they can be used more liberally than in long-term care facilities. The use of a restraint in a prior care setting does not automatically justify its continued use.

Falls in long-term care are a legitimate reason for concern. Statistics cited in the Resident Assessment Protocol for falls say that each year 40 percent of nursing home residents suffer falls and that up to 5 percent result in fractures and 15 percent result in soft tissue injuries such as cuts, abrasions, and bruises. These statistics, as compelling as they are, do not justify automatic use of restraints to prevent falls. Indeed, the protocol provides the warning that restraints can contribute to the occurrence of falls.

No two cases are the same and identical problems may require different solutions from one resident to the next. The following basic assessment points, however, should be looked at in searching for the cause of falls and how to prevent them:

1. Review the apparent causes of falls that have occurred. Did they appear to be caused by loss of balance, sudden weakness, stumbling over objects, or stumbling during turning, bending, or lifting?

2. If dizziness or sudden weakness was involved, have the possible causes been assessed?

3. Have the person's medications been reviewed? Are any of them known to cause sudden drops in blood pressure or dizziness?

4. Is there a history of unstable knee or ankle joints?

5. If falls were related to stumbling, have stumbling hazards and slippery floors been eliminated? Does footwear fit properly and have nonslip soles?

6. If the person normally needs an assistive device for walking such as a cane or walker, was it in use when the falls occurred? Has the person's ability to use the device properly been evaluated?

7. Did poor vision or lighting play a role?

8. Is muscle weakness or joint stiffness causing a gait disturbance? Is physical therapy or restorative therapy a possible solution to that problem?

9. Is the person taking psychoactive medications that can cause very abnormal gait? (See the side effects section of chapter 20, "Powerful Stuff.")

The next most common reason for the use of restraints is "problem behaviors." Among these, aggression or severe agitation is most likely to result in the use of restraint. Problem behaviors are covered in some detail in the chapter on psychoactive medications (chapter 20), where the need to assess the causes of problem behaviors and some alternatives to the use of psychoactive drugs are discussed. We expand on that discussion here.

All long-term care facilities are greatly concerned about aggressive behaviors, which result in possible injury to the resident, to other residents, to staff, and even to visitors in the facility. Preventing such injuries is the facility's responsibility, and taking action to do so is the facility's prerogative. If aggression is frequent and violent, the facility must move quickly and the use of physical restraints may be considered at least temporarily until measures to abate the behavior or remove its cause can be implemented. This requires that the facility provide a high level of supervision for the restrained resident since the more agitated and resistive the resident is, the greater the possibility of injury resulting from struggles against the restraint.

If the behaviors are intense or violent and are frequent or last more than brief periods of time, a psychiatric evaluation may be necessary, perhaps in an inpatient setting. For behaviors that pose a less imminent threat, the facility may be able to arrange for evaluation that will help solve the problem on an outpatient basis. The following checklist can be used by the facility staff in assessing factors that can contribute to "problem behaviors":

1. Do the behaviors occur at a particular time of day?

2. Do they occur only in certain settings, such as the dining room, or around certain other residents or staff? Arranging different seating arrangements or meals in the room may help resolve the problem.

3. Have environmental factors—heat, cold, crowding, noise—been ruled out? Is the light too bright with sharp glare or shadows? Individuals with Alzheimer's disease can be particularly reactive to some of these types of stimulation.

4. Is pain or discomfort a possible factor? Individuals with severe, chronic pain such as that from arthritis require careful pain management. Late or missed doses of pain medication or inadequate assessment of pain can cause real problems for residents with chronic pain.

5. Are there unmet basic needs such as hunger, thirst, or the need for toileting or repositioning?

If the assessment does not lead to a solution, it may be necessary to use a restraint, if only on a temporary basis, until alternatives can be attempted. There are some safety enhancement and alternative devices consumers should be aware of which may be able to be used to solve some of the problems of restraint use. Here are some ideas:

1. Nonslip pads or cushions to help keep the resident from sliding down in a chair, possibly making the use of a lap belt unnecessary, if that's the only concern.

2. A wedge cushion to help keep the resident from sliding down in the chair and assist with posture.

3. Bed or chair alarms.

4. Increased involvement in diversional activities.

5. Use of pillow bolsters for improvement of posture.

6. Gel or foam seat cushions to improve comfort.

7. Increased supervision by staff and volunteers.

8. Frequent walking by staff or creation of safe walking or "wandering" areas.

9. Minimizing noise, bright lights, glare, and other unnecessary sensory stimulation that can cause anxiety or agitated behavior.

10. Use of ambulators, wheeled walkers, or other forms of mobility-assistive devices to keep the resident walking independently as long as possible.

The decision to allow use of a physical restraint can be exceptionally difficult for the spouse or other family member acting as the decision maker. Safety concerns and feelings of guilt about the decision—either way—can be a tremendous burden. However, if the information in this chapter is applied during the decision-making process and afterward, both family and resident can have confidence that every effort has been made to reach the best decision.

22

Freedom from Abuse, Neglect, and Fear

The Right to Safety
and Security

Perhaps nothing is more jarring than the thought of a vulnerable elderly person being made a victim of abuse or mistreatment of any kind. The prospect of it happening is repugnant in itself, but the notion of it happening to a loved one is infuriating. Despite the fact that the OBRA legislation spelled out specific prohibitions against physical, sexual, verbal, and mental abuse and neglect and misappropriation, recent cases and television exposés reveal that there is still the need for vigilance by consumers and enforcement by regulators.

In addition to banning all forms of abuse, neglect, and exploitation, the rules also ban facility practices sometimes referred to as "behavioral management" or "behavioral modification" techniques: corporal punishment and involuntary seclusion.

Fortunately, most long-term care facilities have gotten the message and are budgeting funds for staff education on resident's rights, how to identify, prevent, and report abuse, and stress management. Facilities are, in general, making meaningful efforts in policy development, staff support, and more careful preemployment screening.

Despite progress by the industry in the areas of prevention and education, statistics from the Administration on Aging Long-Term Ombudsman Program Annual Reports for 1995 and 1996 and the Health Care Financing Administration (HCFA) indicate that there are thousands of allegations of abuse, neglect, and misappropriation each year. Table 5 presents data on the number of complaints received by the Long-Term Care Ombudsman program in 29 states reporting full data in 1995 and the same data for 1996, which was the first year the program had uniform data reporting nationwide. Table 6 indicates the number of surveys triggered by allegations of abuse, neglect, misappropriation, resident's rights violations, and poor quality of care from October 1995 to September 1997 based on statistics from the Health Care Financing Administration. These statistics are sobering given the fact that for every incident that made it into these statistics by being detected, reported, and followed up by a survey, an untold number were never spotted, reported, and followed up on with disciplinary action or prosecution.

The statistics from HCFA also reveal that in 1997, survey teams cited 2,390 facilities (13.8 percent of the facilities surveyed) with the inappropriate use

Table 5. Complaints to long-term care ombudsmen, 1995 and 1996

| | Source of Complaint | | | |
| | Nursing facilities | | Board and care | |
Complaint type	1995	1996*	1995	1996*
Residents' rights				
Abuse, neglect, or exploitation	6,128	13,469	915	3,701
Access to information	1,455	3,120	189	942
Admit, transfer, discharge, or eviction	4,533	8,192	565	1,550
Autonomy, choice, rights, privacy	7,978	14,383	1,247	3,205
Financial, property	4,493	7,745	1,247	2,251
Category totals	24,587	46,909	3,712	11,649
Resident care				
Quality of care	21,592	37,707	1,815	5,609
Rehabilitation, maintenance of function	3,226	5,004	222	542
Restraint use, chemical or physical	1,127	1,682	206	349
Category totals	25,954	44,392	2,243	6,500
Quality of life				
Activities and social services	2,890	4,370	369	1,000
Dietary	6,994	10,533	1,229	2,579
Environment	7,896	12,382	1,756	3,337
Category totals	17,780	27,285	3,354	6,916
Administration				
Policies, procedure, attitude	1,420	2,915	570	1,360
Staffing	6,327	11,121	715	2,133
Category totals	7,747	14,036	1,285	3,493
Not against a facility				
Certification or licensing agency	175	725	39	165
State Medicaid agency	690	1,770	66	194
System or other	5,518	9,563	1,017	2,743
Category totals	6,383	12,058	1,122	3,102
Grand totals	82,442	144,680	11,716	31,660

*1996 data are the first reported by all states using the same system. 1995 data from the Administration on Aging based on reports from 29 states providing full data. Of these complaints, 72 percent were verified and 60 percent were resolved to the satisfaction of the complainant. The 23 remaining jurisdictions reporting (using a different system than the one used for the 1995 data reported above) had 123,341 complaints, of which 77 percent were resolved or partially resolved. Of those, 82 percent were about nursing homes and 10 percent were about board and care or similar types of facilities.

Table 6. Allegations reported to HCFA against nursing facilities

Allegation	Number reported, October 1, 1995– September 31, 1996	Number reported, October 1, 1996– September 31, 1997
Resident abuse	1,173	707*
Resident neglect	446	397*
Violation of resident rights	515	360*
Poor quality of care	1,643	1,300*
Misuse of resident funds or property	38	25*
Total[a]	3,815	2,789*

Note: The number of facilities against which complaints were filed between October 1, 1995, and September 31, 1996, was 4,540; between October 1, 1996, and September 31, 1997, it was 3,305.*

*Data were obtained from HCFA on October 20, 1997, and may not capture all pending allegations received by that agency after that date but alleged to have occurred before September 31, 1997.

of physical restraints as a result of their regular survey.[1] They also cited 257 facilities (1.49 percent) for failing to uphold the resident's right to be free from abuse and 836 facilities (4.84 percent) for employing persons who had been found guilty of committing acts of abuse in the past. In addition, 2,299 facilities had been cited (13.3 percent of those facilities surveyed) for failure to uphold the residents' right to personal dignity and 1,175 (6.8 percent) were cited for failure to ensure personal privacy.

Considering that these surveys are, at best, annual events spanning a few days up to perhaps two weeks, it becomes very clear that there is a significant amount of work yet to be done in long-term care facilities to improve quality of care. To be sure, the majority of people receiving care in *skilled nursing facilities* and *nursing facilities* that are covered by the inspections discussed above will have good, appropriate care. But among those people whose needs are served by the nation's long-term care facilities (SNFs and NFs), even a few exceptions are unacceptable.

In an age when state budgets rarely provide sufficient funds for conducting enforcement surveys, it is clear the state survey teams cannot do the job alone. The answer lies in an informed public: the *residents in long-term care facilities*

and their decision makers, friends, advocates, and families need to know what to look for and what to do. Family members, friends, and decision makers of nursing home residents should visit frequently and at varying times of the day. They should be vigilant for signs of abuse, neglect, mistreatment and misappropriation, poor quality of care, poor quality of life, or any infringement of residents' rights. Finally, they should be outspoken and direct in reporting these types of concerns to facility management. Consumers and their family members or decision makers should be uncompromising in demanding that the standards described in this book be met.

In addition to the rules in OBRA, which hold the *facility* accountable for incidents of abuse, states have enacted legislation to increase the penalties to *individuals* found to have committed abuse. In a number of states, committing abuse to a nursing home resident has been made a felony and penalties can be imposed in addition to the federally required step of reporting the abuse to the state nurse aide registry. When such a finding is reported to a state registry, it *should* effectively close the door to any future employment in a nursing home. This is because OBRA prohibits nursing homes from employing an aide with a finding in the state's registry of abuse or misappropriation. But the

1. 42 CFR 488.308 requires that facilities be subject to a standard survey no later than 15 months from the date of their last survey and that the average interval between surveys should not be more than 12 months. A complaint survey can occur at any time. A survey team generally consists of registered nurses, social workers, dietician, hygienist, or others with specialized background. The number and mix of skills can vary based on the size of the facility and the type of survey.

registry is effective only if all facilities report all findings of abuse or misappropriation and all facilities perform the required query to the registry before extending an offer of employment. As the foregoing statistics show, nearly 5 percent of the facility surveys resulted in the discovery that people with a finding of abuse or misappropriation on the state registry were still employed in nursing homes.

■
Types of Abuse Defined

OBRA defines abuse as

> *willful infliction of injury, unreasonable confinement, intimidation or punishment, with resulting physical harm or pain or mental anguish, or deprivation by an individual, including a caretaker, of goods or services that are necessary to attain or maintain physical, mental or psychosocial well-being. This presumes that instances of abuse of all residents, even those in a coma, cause physical harm, or pain or mental anguish.*
>
> *[42 CFR Sec. 483.13(b)(c)]*

This broad definition works to the advantage of residents or decision makers only if they know and understand it. It has sweeping application to facility practices, case management, and resident quality of life.

The use of denial or deprivation of goods or services or involuntary seclusion of a resident as a method of discipline or punishment constitutes abuse if it causes any physical harm, mental anguish, or intimidation or if it results in denial of anything necessary for the maintenance of physical, mental, or psychosocial well-being—for example, the facility allows staff to deny food to a resident for "misbehaving," or the staff ignores the resident's call light even though they may have the time to answer. It could also include not providing incontinent care or skin care and

exercise for a resident in retaliation for some alleged offense the resident may have committed.

The following definitions are from "Guidance to Surveyors—Long-Term Care Facilities" (HCFA, July 1995).

INVOLUNTARY SECLUSION

This is defined as any confinement of a resident to his or her room or separation from his or her room or other residents against the resident's will or without the consent of the resident's decision maker. This definition *does not* include the use of short-term seclusion of a resident on an emergency basis to prevent injury to the resident or others because of violent behavior. It is allowed only during the time the threatening behavior persists and only long enough for the facility to develop an appropriate care plan.

Consumers should ask the facility they're dealing with for a copy of its policy on dealing with combative or aggressive behavioral emergencies.

VERBAL ABUSE

The definition of verbal abuse is given in the surveyor's guidelines:

Any use of oral, written or gestured language that willfully includes disparaging and derogatory terms to residents or their families, or within their hearing distance, regardless of their age, ability to comprehend, or disability. Examples of verbal abuse include, but are not limited to threats of harm, saying things to frighten a resident, such as telling a resident that she will never be able to see her family again.

This definition leaves a great deal of room for interpretation and it could apply to a great many situations. Some remarks that do not meet this definition can nonetheless hurt residents or their families deeply. Some remarks, by their *content* only, appear not to meet the definition of verbal abuse but, if viewed in the *way* the words are spoken, can be verbal abuse. For example, simple messages spoken in an ominous or intimidating way could meet the definition. In such cases, it may be necessary to construe the message in light of the effect it had on the resident.

SEXUAL ABUSE

Sexual abuse "includes, but is not limited to, sexual harassment, sexual coercion or sexual assault." This succinct definition would seem to say it all, but in a setting where male or female caregivers can be called on to care for both male and female residents, the opportunities for prohibited conduct occur dozens of times per day. This type of activity is both abhorrent and criminal, but what is worse, it can be very hard to detect, especially if the victim is comatose or unable to communicate.

Prevention is the best medicine for dealing with all forms of abuse. Part of the effort to prevent individuals who may commit such abuse from ever having the opportunity is due diligence in the hiring process. This includes the mandatory nurse aide registry check on each nurse aide prior to the offer of employment and, in a growing number of states, a mandatory criminal background check. Thanks to new information technology, in many states it is possible to obtain information on felony convictions for a nominal fee. Surprisingly, such background checks are not required by OBRA.

Ask the facility you are using or considering whether criminal background checks are required in your state and if not, whether the facility itself requires criminal background checks prior to all new hires starting work in the facility. It is something to consider when selecting a facility to care for a vulnerable loved one.

PHYSICAL ABUSE

Physical abuse includes "hitting, slapping, pinching and kicking. It also includes controlling behavior through corporal punishment." Although it's not stated explicitly in OBRA, it would probably be safe to extend this definition to include any deliberate act intended to cause pain or harm whether there is physical injury or not. Thus the category includes deliberately applying a restraint too tightly, deliberate roughness during transfers or repositioning, or using force to administer treatment that is not essential to save the resident's life.

It is up to the facility to thoroughly investigate any allegation of abuse and to report that allegation to the appropriate licensing authority. If you suspect or know of an incident of abuse, report it to the facility at once. Generally, the report is taken by the facility social services staff or social services director, but it can be made to any nursing supervisor, the assistant director of nursing, the director of nursing, or the administrator. The facility must take your report in confidence and act immediately to prevent further abuse from occurring. It is a good idea to ask the facility for a copy of its policy in dealing with abuse if it is not routinely provided during the admission process. The facility must inform you of the outcome of the investigation.

MENTAL ABUSE

This includes but is not limited to "humiliation, harassment, threats of punishment or deprivation." As with sexual abuse, the opportunities to commit mental abuse occur on a daily basis. For an already confused, agitated resident, finding words to express the anguish that results from this type of offense can be impossible. Detecting signs that it is occurring can likewise be very difficult. Nevertheless, if you have concerns that an incident has happened, or that such conduct is occurring or may occur, discuss these concerns with the facility staff. State your reasons and work with the facility to ensure that your concerns are fully addressed.

Taunting, ridicule, embarrassment, and threats of any kind will not be tolerated by any reputable facility.

NEGLECT

Neglect is defined in the guidance to surveyors as "the failure to provide goods and services necessary to avoid physical harm, mental anguish or mental illness. Neglect occurs on an individual basis when a resident does not receive care in one or more areas (e.g., the lack of frequent monitoring for a resident known to be incontinent, resulting in being left to lie in urine or feces."

Neglect tends to leave footprints behind. Watch for these telltale occurrences that are completely preventable:

1. Skin breakdown.

2. The persistent odor of urine or feces about a resident.

3. Dirt under the resident's fingernails; nails left long and untrimmed.

4. The resident's clothing constantly stained, dirty, or not put on (i.e., the resident is often left in a hospital gown instead of being appropriately dressed during the day).

5. Dentures not put in, even at mealtime, whether the resident desires them in or not.

6. Weight loss not attributable to any medical cause.

7. Persistently unkempt, ungroomed hair.

8. Poor dental and oral health.

9. Glasses put on with lenses so filthy they cannot be seen through.

10. Residents left sitting alone for long periods of time.

These are but a few indicators of what could be a pattern of neglect, especially if they happen together and happen often.

Neglect has a perilous cohort that is referred to as *endangerment.* Though this is not included in the rules covering neglect, it could be thought of as any form of neglect, an act or omission that places the resident's health or even life in jeopardy. Examples include leaving a confused resident alone in a wheelchair at the top of a stairway or leaving a confused and weakened resident who requires assistance to stand and transfer alone in a tub full of water or sitting unattended on a commode.

MISAPPROPRIATION OF RESIDENT PROPERTY

The surveyor's guidelines define this as "the patterned or deliberate misplacement, exploitation, or wrongful, temporary or permanent use of a resident's belongings or money without the resident's consent." Most facilities strongly advise residents to place their valuables in the facility safe or, better, not bring them to the facility at all. That is good advice, but some belongings bring a degree of comfort and remembrance, which makes them all the more precious. For the resident likely to need an extended or permanent stay, such items may be of great importance. Some people want to keep some cash with them in their room, even though there are usually few ways to spend it within the facility. These cases present the unavoidable risk that the loss of such items or money may occur, even in the best facilities. There is the risk of theft by a staff member as well as the risk that other residents may take such items, convinced that the items belong to them. Though it can be a difficult thing to do, a good rule of thumb to follow is to never keep anything in a resident room that you could not bear to lose.

Misappropriation is a crime of opportunity. Denying access to items of value denies the opportunity. When a resident cannot do without certain valuable items, it may be useful to photograph, catalog, and somehow mark each for identification. If a valuable item disappears from your room in a long-term care facility, report the loss to the facility social services staff at once. Give all the identifying information you can, including photographs if you have them and a detailed description listing identifying marks or inscriptions and their locations. A very important piece of information to provide, if you can, is the time when the item may have disappeared or when the loss was discovered.

Frequently when an item disappears, a caregiver is held responsible. The best way a nursing assistant can avoid any suspicion is to *never take anything* of value from a resident, even if it is offered as a gift or a "tip." And the resident, analogously, should never offer a newspaper, a book, jewelry, keepsakes, anything. Taking—or giving—anything can invite disaster and creates the possibility of an allegation of misappropriation, even if that was not the case. Taking the offer of a gift or tip is prohibited in most facilities and there can never be an expectation by staff for such gifts to be given.

All of these aspects of the protections of residents' rights are extremely important to people living in a long-term care facility and to their families and/or decision makers. Consumers should ask the facility for information concerning policies on prevention of abuse, neglect, and misappropriation and procedures for dealing with each.

If an incident occurs which you feel fits a definition of abuse given here and your report of the incident to the facility does not bring action, you may wish to report the problem to the office of the state long-term care ombudsman (see appendix J) or the state survey agency (see appendix I). Information on how to reach these agencies also must be provided to you by the facility upon your request and such information must be displayed in the facility. The state department of health or social services should provide referral for specific types of problems as well.

For additional information on the facility's performance record with regard to quality-of-care and abuse issues, ask to see the most recent survey reports and any reports of complaint surveys that may have occurred. The office of the state long-term care ombudsman may also have useful information on these topics (see appendix J for the ombudsman's office in your state).

In addition to this information, the facility must make available to you information about the plan of correction it has developed to address any deficiencies (the term used to describe noncompliance with regulations) noted by the survey team. The facility must keep a copy of its most recent survey report in a location accessible to the residents and the facility must post information about the availability of the report in the facility. Another good report to ask for is the On-Line Survey Certification and Report (OSCAR) 3, a summary of the citations issued against the facility over the past few years, which quickly reveals the types of citation issued and whether there have been repeat citations for the same deficiencies. The facility may *not* edit or alter the content of these reports in any way. You may also access the most recent survey information at HCFA's Nursing Home Compare Internet website at: http://www.medicare.gov./nursing/home.asp.

■

TECHNIQUES THAT ARE NOT CONSIDERED ABUSE

OBRA recognizes that there are times when the facility may need to employ techniques for short-term emergency control of aggressive behavior that would, under other circumstances, be considered unacceptable.

INVOLUNTARY SECLUSION

This is not considered abuse to a resident when it is done to prevent the individual from injuring himself or herself or others as the result of violent behavior. Every effort must be made to treat the cause of the behavior and end the seclusion as soon as possible. The facility must assess the behavior, seek less restrictive means of dealing with it, modify the care plan to reflect the changes necessary to treat the behavior, and involve the resident (to the extent possible) and/or the decision maker in making informed choices about the use of seclusion.

RESTRAINTS

Physical restraints and psychoactive medications may be used on a short-term basis in emergency situations such as those just described, but the rules discussed in the chapters on each still apply. Where physical restraints are concerned, if the behavior is so agitated that the resident struggles against the physical restraint and there is a danger of injury, the facility must provide adequate supervision, one-on-one if need be, to prevent such injury until that likelihood passes or it becomes necessary to transfer the resident to an appropriate setting.

The use of physical restraint against the person's wishes is allowed for the administration of medical treatment necessary to treat a life-threatening condition and the provision of the treatment does not conflict with the resident's advance directive.

WHAT HAPPENS WHEN YOU FILE A COMPLAINT ABOUT SUSPECTED ABUSE?

Perhaps the most important thing to know about filing a complaint is knowing what *must not* happen as a result of that complaint. The facility cannot act in reprisal or discriminate in any way against the resident filing the complaint or in whose behalf the complaint was filed. This is one of the fundamental residents' rights in OBRA [42 CFR Sec. 483.10(f)]. The identity of the complainant must be held in confidence.

The resident also has the right to expect that the facility will act *promptly* on any grievance or complaint—not just those related to the facility or its staff, but on complaints arising out of the conduct of other residents as well. When the complaint is about suspected abuse, the facility must take decisive action to prevent the possibility that further abuse could occur. The facility must investigate promptly and keep the resident and/or family or decision maker informed of the steps taken and progress made in dealing with the situation.

The facility should also report all confirmed allegations of abuse to its respective licensing offices, usually within a time frame set by the state. The allegation should be reported by the facility, even if its internal investigation has not yet been completed. The state licensing and certification office may conduct an independent investigation into the causes of any complaint.

23

Survey and Enforcement

TOUGH NEW RULES TO ENSURE
THAT LONG-TERM CARE FACILITIES
PROVIDE CONSISTENT,
HIGH-QUALITY CARE

On July 1, 1995, new survey and certification rules went into effect for long-term care facilities. The rules were designed to address the need for consistent, ongoing quality of care and service. The rules are intended to ensure that any problems identified in those areas are quickly corrected, that problems *stay* corrected once they are corrected, and that residents receive all the care and services they need; finally, they provide survey agencies with potent new tools to enforce compliance.

Nursing facilities (NFs) and skilled nursing facilities (SNFs) must be inspected or surveyed at least every 15 months by the state survey agency. A facility may be surveyed more often than that, but not less often. Survey agencies are required to conduct surveys as often as necessary to get a facility into compliance with the rules and keep it there.

Surveys are unannounced and in addition to the annual survey, the facility may be subject to inspection following a change of ownership, administrator, or director of nursing or if the facility has been placed under the control of a management firm. The survey agency may conduct a survey to ensure that such changes do not have an adverse impact on the quality of care.

The survey agency may also conduct an unannounced special inspection based on a consumer complaint. A complaint may be a report of any kind of improper or inadequate care, resident mistreatment, or abuse. The complaint can originate with a resident; family member, decision maker, or advocate; a facility staff member; a physician; the state long-term care ombudsman; the local social services office or health department; or anyone having knowledge of such infractions.

Although the survey agency will ask the identity of the person making the complaint, if that person chooses to remain anonymous, the complaint will still be investigated. Complaints may be made either orally or in writing. See appendixes I and J for the addresses and phone numbers of the state survey agencies and the long-term care ombudsman's offices.

Survey rules previously assigned a higher level of importance to certain requirements, implying that some requirements were more important than others. Under the survey rules enacted in 1995, all requirements are viewed as equally important. All deficiencies (the term used by survey agencies for any failure to meet a requirement) are cited in the facility's survey report. The survey rules introduce a system for evaluating the scope and severity of the deficiencies in order to determine whether the facility is in *substantial compliance* with the rules, or, if not, to aid in determining the appropriate enforcement action.

The system uses a scoring grid that assigns four *levels of severity* that categorize the deficiency by the level of harm that has or may result from the deficiency. The system defines the *scope* (how many residents the deficiency is likely to affect) by three categories. Based on the combination of scope and severity, the deficiency then is placed on the scoring matrix (see figure 10) to determine whether the facility is in substantial compliance or is so far out of compliance that it is providing substandard quality of care and to determine the remedies the survey team may recommend to the regional office, which has the final authority in assessing penalties or imposing corrective actions.

The phrase **substandard quality of care** has a specific meaning in the long-term care facility survey. A facility will be deemed to have provided substandard quality of care if it is found to have one or more deficiencies in any of the requirements in any of three broad categories:

1. Resident behavior and facility practices (Sec. 483.13),

2. Quality of life (Sec. 483.15), or

3. Quality of care (Sec. 483.25).

Any of the deficiencies would have to constitute one or more of the following:

1. Immediate jeopardy to health or safety.

2. A pattern of or widespread actual harm.

3. Widespread potential for more than minimal harm, with no actual harm having occurred and posing less than immediate jeopardy to resident health or safety.

The rules also make a range of remedies available to the state survey agency, which could be used to compel compliance with the regulations. Those remedies include:

1. **Directed plan of correction.** If the facility is in substantial compliance but has some deficiencies that lack the scope and severity to be considered substandard quality of care, the facility will be required to write its own plan of correction (PoC). If, however, the facility was found to have deficiencies that are serious enough to require specific actions in a specific time frame to ensure the problems are corrected and stay corrected, the survey agency may dictate the plan of correction and the schedule for its implementation.

2. **Directed in-service training.** When the survey agency determines that staff education is necessary to correct deficiencies, it may specify the training program for the facility and require that the facility's staff complete the training.

3. **State monitoring.** To prevent harm or further harm from resulting from deficient practices in a facility, the survey agency may place in the facility a **monitor,** an individual with appropriate qualifications to oversee the actions of the facility to correct its problems. State monitoring is required if the facility has been found to have provided substandard quality of care on three consecutive standard surveys. It is available as an option to the survey agency if the facility has had a poor compliance history, if the situation in the facility may get worse before it gets better, if the deficiencies are serious enough to pose a threat for immediate jeopardy to the residents' health or safety, if the facility is unable or unwilling to make adequate correction, or, if the facility has been ordered closed due to the magnitude of the problems, to oversee the transfer of the facility's residents to other facilities.

4. **Denial of payment.** Denial of payment for new admissions may be imposed when the facility is found to have failed to achieve substantial compliance with the

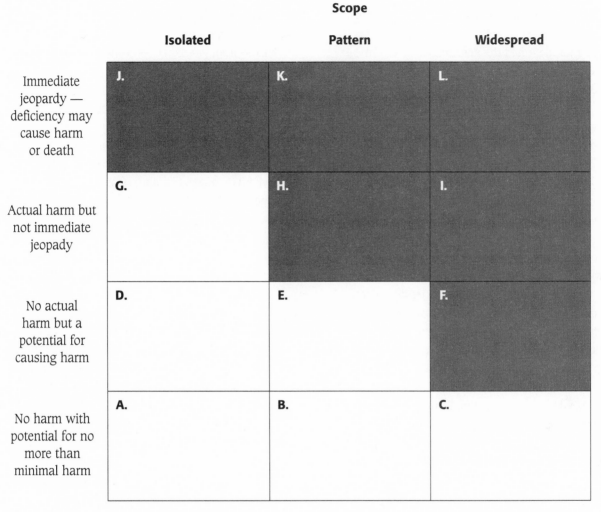

The facility is in substantial compliance if deficiencies fall into the white boxes of the matrix. Substandard quality of care exists if they are in the shaded boxes.

requirements. This remedy may be imposed when the facility fails to make a serious effort to get into compliance, for example, it fails to carry out its own plan of correction to correct its deficiencies. Denial of payment for new admissions is mandatory when the facility is still not in substantial compliance three months after the survey that identified the noncompliance or if the facility is found to have provided substandard quality care by three consecutive standard surveys. Denial of payment for all Medicare and Medicaid residents may be imposed. Since this would be a serious penalty for a facility to face, it is reserved for very serious situations, or when lesser remedies have not achieved compliance.

5. **Civil money penalties.** The facility may be required to pay a fine officially referred to as a civil money penalty (CMP). The CMP may be imposed if the facility is found to have had "egregious past noncompliance." On the low end, the facility could face fines from $50 per day up to $3,000 per day when the deficiencies do not impose jeopardy but either have caused harm or have the potential for doing more than minimal harm to the residents. For cases where immediate jeopardy exists, or where deficiencies serious enough to have elicited previous civil money penalties are repeated, civil money penalties may be imposed ranging from $3,050 per day up to $10,000 per day. "Per day" means each day that the survey agency is able to document that the deficient practice existed in the facility.

6. **Temporary management.** The facility may be placed under temporary management when the survey agency is convinced that the current facility management is incapable of making the necessary corrections to bring the facility into compliance. This rather drastic step may be considered when the facility's deficiencies pose immediate jeopardy to the residents or have actually caused widespread harm to resident health or safety. Temporary management may also be put in place to oversee the closure of the facility.

7. **Transfer of residents or transfer of residents with facility closure.** In very serious cases, the survey agency or the Health Care Financing Administration (HCFA) may order the Medicare and Medicaid residents in a facility to be transferred to other facilities. This would require the state Medicaid agency to act as well. This may be either permanent or temporary until the facility makes corrections sufficient to deal with its quality problems. In cases where the order is permanent, it is likely that the facility is being terminated from participation in the Medicare and Medicaid programs and will be closed.

8. **Termination of provider agreements.** The termination of provider agreements with a facility means that the facility cannot receive payment for any Medicare or Medicaid resident beyond a certain date. In a case where the noncompliance poses immediate jeopardy to the resident's safety or health, the termination procedure must be completed within 23 days of the last day of the survey which identified the immediate jeopardy. If the facility can prove it has removed the immediate jeopardy prior to that time, the facility may be granted a reprieve from the termination process, but it will have to remain in substantial compliance on an ongoing basis to avoid restarting the termination process.

The rules also provide for an **informal dispute resolution** process, which the facility can follow if it disagrees with the findings of the survey process. The facility may use the informal dispute resolution *only* to present facts that would contradict the findings and subsequent citations of deficiencies made by the survey team. The facility will not get more than one hearing to do this and the request for a hearing cannot be used to delay the imposition of remedies that the state may have ordered.

Once the survey is complete and any informal dispute resolution is done, the facility must then implement its plans to correct any deficiencies within a set time frame. If the facility is in substantial compliance with the rules, it will be granted some latitude in the amount of time that it has for implementing the plan, but it must submit the plan of correction to the state within 10 days of receiving the survey report (statement of deficiencies). After that, the facility must carry out its plan and report that it has done so by sending the state survey agency a notification called an "allegation of compliance." This can be the same document as the plan of correction.

If the state survey agency accepts the plan of correction and allegation of compliance, it may then make a **verification visit** on an unannounced basis to ensure that the facility is, in fact, in compliance. If it finds that the facility is not in compliance or it rejects the plan of correction/allegation of compliance, it may choose to impose remedies of its own.

The survey rules also reinforce the public's right to know the outcomes of long-term care surveys. OBRA rules (42 CFR Sec. 488.325) require that the state survey agency, the Medicaid agency, and HCFA each must disclose at the public's request any of the following documents:

1. HCFA form 2567, which includes both the survey statement of deficiencies (SoD) and the facility's plan of correction (PoC). When you request a copy of a survey report, you must specify the year or years of the reports that you wish to obtain. If you obtain copies of reports and information appears to have been deleted, it may be because the example the surveyor cited has been withdrawn as the result of the informal dispute resolution process. If that is the case, there should be a note written in to that effect.

2. Provider comments that may have been documented.

3. Notification letters to the facility if its plan of correction was rejected or of failure to implement remedies that may have been imposed.

4. Notices of termination from the Medicare or Medicaid programs.

5. Statistical data on the facility's performance, such as the OSCAR 3 and 4 reports (see appendix P).

6. Final results of appeals or informal dispute resolution proceedings.

7. Medicare and Medicaid cost reports.

8. The names of individuals with ownership interests in the facility. This will include the names of any individuals who have been found guilty of criminal violations of Medicare or Medicaid laws.

Requests for information should be in writing and there will generally be a nominal charge for producing copies of the documents requested. The information must be provided no later than 14 days after it has been made available to the facility itself and may be disclosed to the public the day after it is made available to the facility if the survey agency deems that it is appropriate to do so. The survey agency will also provide survey and appeal information to the state long-term care ombudsman's office. In the case of Medicaid participating facilities, the survey agency also will routinely provide access to survey information to the state Medicaid Fraud Control Unit (MFCU).

When there is a finding of substandard quality of care, the facility is required to provide the state survey agency with a list of the names of residents in the facility to whom such a finding was made and the name and address of the attending physician for each of those residents. The survey agency will then notify each physician of the residents involved in the finding of substandard quality of care and will notify the state board responsible for licensing the facility's administrator. These notifications will go out within 20 days of the survey agency receiving the information from the facility.

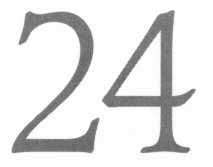

Going Home and Staying Home

DISCHARGE PLANNING AND
ALTERNATIVES TO NURSING
HOME CARE

The rapid growth of home and community-based care and supportive services over the past decade has opened new options in meeting people's needs. According to the Centers for Disease Control report called *Advance Data* (Number 280, January 23, 1997), home health care agencies surged ahead of nursing homes as care providers for individuals over the age of 65. The report states that the number of people being cared for by home health agencies per 1,000 people over the age of 65 was greater than the number in nursing homes nationwide by 1994. Home health agencies provided care to 41.6 out of every 1,000 people over the age 65 while nursing homes provided care to 41.3.

The trend toward home health care continues to grow, despite a federal effort in 1997 to curb increases in spending on home health and an executive order to curb the growth of new home health branch offices. Meanwhile, the utilization of nursing home beds continues to slowly fall. However, this trend may not last much longer as the number of individuals over the age 65 as a percentage of the nation's total population continues to grow and the number of people over the age of 85 also grows. This is the age group most likely to require the services of a nursing home.

According to the *Hoechst Marion Roussel Institutional Digest 1996,* the home care industry has nearly tripled in size since 1986, when there were 5,250 agencies in operation. By 1995, that number had grown to 15,037. As is the case with nursing homes, the largest entities providing home health services are for-profit corporations. According to the digest, the 12 largest providers of home health services in the nation were private, for-profit corporations.

Home health agencies can vary somewhat in the level of services they are capable of providing and the number of hours of services they can staff. In general, home health services provide skilled nursing (RN, LPN, nurse practitioner) services, home health aides, and therapy services such as physical, respiratory, speech, and occupational therapy. Medical social services are also provided. These services are generally covered by Medicare and/or Medicaid for those who qualify. Medicare imposes a number of restrictions on when it will pay for home health services (see chapter 2, "Paying for Care"). Most state Medicaid programs will require a prior authorization before services are covered and, unlike Medicare, there are income and asset eligibility requirements that apply.

Some agencies may have personal care workers, home-makers, and companions, who do not provide health-related services but assist with bathing, dressing, personal grooming, housekeeping, shopping, and the like. These services are not covered by Medicare, but in some cases may be covered by Medicaid or other state or county funding programs.

In some locations, individuals who need assistance only with nonmedical care or routine daily living tasks may be provided with supportive services through county or state-run programs. Excellent examples of this type of service are found in the state of Wisconsin, whose Community Options Program (COP) and Community Integration Program (CIP) are designed to provide services in the community to elderly or disabled individuals who otherwise may have required nursing home care.

Since about 68 percent of the people who are admitted to nursing homes are admitted directly from an acute care hospital, the hospital discharge planners play an important role in helping to decide whether to use a nursing home or a home health agency for any subsequent care that is required. The physician plays a defining role in the care planning process, and if the decision to use home health and community-based services or a nursing home is a close call, the physician will generally favor nursing home placement, where the patient's safety as well as care needs are likely to be best served in a setting with round-the-clock staffing. Still, the individual's preferences must be considered, and if comprehensive services are available in the person's home setting, it may be possible to forgo nursing home placement.

There may be times when a person who has not been in the hospital has a health problem that can be addressed effectively with home health services and supportive services. In this case, the physician and the individual (or the decision maker) play the lead roles in creating the care plan. Medicare will pay for home health services and, unlike the nursing home benefit, there is no requirement for a qualifying hospital stay before home health services are covered. (See chapter 2, "Home Health Services" section.)

For assistance locating home and community-based services in your area, contact your county department of human services or the state agency on aging (see appendix G) or consult the yellow pages under "Nurses."

DISCHARGE PLANNING

For most people, the very thought of ever being admitted to a nursing home is abhorrent—often because of the conviction that once a person goes into a nursing home, the door is closed forever. However, more than 1.2 million people are *discharged* from nursing homes each year, and the number is growing.

The concept of the nursing home placement as being automatically permanent is fading rapidly. These days, more and more people go to nursing facilities for convalescent stays that involve wound care, rehabilitation, therapy, or continued complex medical care. When these services are no longer necessary, the individual is often discharged home. If the patient will still need nursing care, but only on an intermittent basis, he or she may be referred to a home health agency for assistance in continuing to recover at home.

The time to begin discussing the discharge plan with the nursing home staff and the physician is at the point of admission to the facility. The length of time a person will need to be in the nursing home will vary, depending on the reasons the individual was admitted in the first place and how well recovery goes.

During the assessment process, the nursing facility staff will estimate the length of stay required for each person admitted in Section Q of the Minimum Data Set (MDS; see chapter 9). Section Q also asks if the person being admitted indicates a preference to return to the community and whether there is a "support person who is positive towards discharge."

These questions can actually be difficult to answer during the admission process. Dramatic changes may occur during the nursing home stay, and they may alter the answers, both for the person being admitted and for the support person. For example, a spouse who is the resident's only support person at home may *not* be able to express support for discharge back to the family home if the patient is in a condition that poses overwhelming care needs at the time of admission to the nursing home. Further, the spouse may not be aware at that point of what, if any, supportive community services are available in the locality.

However, in 20 or 30 days, the resident's condition may have improved and the spouse may have been able to discover that many services provided in the nursing home can be obtained at home from various local agencies. This can alter the answers to the questions in Section Q and, more important, alter the speed of the operation of the discharge plan.

Nursing homes cannot always accurately estimate the length of a stay in the facility. Statistics from the state of Wisconsin, for example, reveal that nursing homes there estimated that discharge would occur within three months of the date of admission 31 percent of the time. However, the *actual* number of discharges that occurred within three months was only 8 percent.

For all of the foregoing reasons, it is important for residents themselves (when they have the capacity to do so) as well as their family members or decision makers to stay abreast of how things are going in the nursing facility and help advance the discharge planning process.

The tendency on the part of nursing homes can be to follow the required minimums where care planning and discharge planning meeting frequency is concerned. This will lead to the care planning sessions to occur soon after admission and not later than every 90 days thereafter. The resident or decision makers can help advance the process by taking an active role in staying informed on the current care needs and conditions and in the discharge planning process.

■
WHO MAKES THE DISCHARGE DECISION?

As with all decisions pertaining to an individual's health care and treatment, the individual makes the decisions. Unless the individual has been found to be incapable of making those decisions (see chapter 17, "Advance Direc-

tives"), the individual's preference about time of discharge should be honored by the facility. In the case of an individual who *has* been found to be incapable of making care and treatment decisions, the person's designated decision maker must make the decision.

In either case, the decision must be based on the physician's advice, the facility's input, the availability of necessary services in the community, and the person's best interests. The decision to leave the nursing home may seem to be a simple thing at first, but it really can be a lot more complicated than just deciding to leave.

After noting that you, as the consumer, have the authority to make the discharge decision basically no matter what anyone says (as long as you are competent to make the decision), it also must be said that taking that decision too soon can be self-defeating. Leaving a facility too soon can lead to complications that may lead to readmission or slower recovery.

The decision should be made the same way as any other care and treatment decision is made—that is, based on all the facts. It should be a reasoned, well-thought-out decision. That means that if discharge earlier than is recommended by the attending physician and the facility discharge planning staff is desired, there should be a thorough discussion of care needs and medical conditions affecting the decision *before* leaving the facility. Leaving against your physician's advice is called "leaving AMA" (against medical advice). It is within a person's right to leave a facility this way, assuming the individual has not been protectively placed by a court of law, but it is generally a bad idea. The decision to leave AMA may be based on emotional factors, so it is always a good idea to consult fully with the physician about the consequences of such an action before going ahead. If this is the decision even after the possible consequences are understood, the facility and the physician still have an obligation to help plan care services to meet the individual's needs at home.

The length of your stay may be determined to a great extent by your payer source. For individuals covered by commercial or Medicare HMOs the tendency may be toward shorter stays than in the past. The 100-day benefit for skilled nursing under Medicare, which is described in chapter 2, may not be fully utilized.

Nevertheless, you have a right to have a say on the issue of discharge planning whether you are in an HMO plan or not. If you are in a Medicare HMO, you should be supplied with some specific information about your rights as a Medicare beneficiary and whom to contact if you feel that you are being discharged from the facility too early.

In any case, the facility must work with your insurer, your physician, and you to make sure that there is continuity of care. This means that discharge of a resident is not the end of the facility's responsibility. If the person being discharged continues to have health care needs, such as therapy, or nursing care needs as well as the need for supportive community services or social services, the facility must assist in making arrangements for such services.

Throughout this book we have examined the effectiveness of the nursing home reforms known as OBRA. From a consumer's perspective, evidence suggests mixed results at best. In late 1996, Congress commissioned a report to evaluate the following:

1. The use of private accreditation systems to replace the current inspection system (called deeming).

2. The use of regulatory and nonregulatory incentives to improve nursing home care.

3. The effectiveness of the current certification and survey process.

The report was prepared by Abt Associates, a contractor acting as an independent evaluator. (It is available on the HCFA website.) The following conclusions were made on each of the three approaches:

With respect to granting deeming authority (the most likely organization to perform this function being JCAHO), evidence indicates that as presently structured, offering the deeming option to facilities would place many residents at serious risk. In contrast, the HCFA survey as typically implemented with all its flaws, identifies many serious problems, allows less time for problems to remain uncorrected, and verifies compliance by an actual revisit as compared to JCAHO.

An assessment of the second strategy, various regulatory incentives and non-regulatory nursing home quality improvement initiatives, provided little to no evidence that these efforts are effective and could supplant the normal survey process. At best, we would have to conclude that the evidence is not in.

With respect to the third strategy, the existing system of survey and certification, evidence was produced that the OBRA '87 reforms implemented in October 1990 resulted in improved resident outcomes. Also, there is some suggestive but inconclusive evidence that the more recent enforcement provisions resulted in improvements in resident outcomes, although many of the enforcement processes we examined are not working as intended. There is a concern that several States never or very rarely cite a substandard care deficiency.

The evidence examined in this study is supportive not only of regulation as the primary bulwark for quality assurance, but that enforcement needs to be more vigorously applied among the States. Although a thorough discussion of possible solutions to redress the problems in the Federal survey and certification process is beyond the scope of this report to Congress, the Department is currently in the process of identifying improvements to the current system.

As has happened in the past, the role of informed, empowered consumers has been overlooked in the context of the report and in the role of quality improvement. The simple fact is that while the report calls for more vigorous inspection, Congress has not supported that call with more vigorous financial support for the inspection process. Even if it did, the report suggests some considerable weaknesses in the survey system that are not going to change.

In July 1998, Donna Shalala, secretary of Health and Human Services (HHS), announced a nursing home initiative. The initiative includes a number of approaches to improve care. They include:

1. Tougher inspection and sanction policies that will cause nursing homes with repeat violations of the standards that result in harm to residents to face sanctions without a grace period and without the ability to avoid the sanctions.

2. More frequent inspections for nursing homes with repeated violations while maintaining the current frequency of inspection for all other facilities.

3. Less predictable survey schedules and a requirement for surveys to occur on weekends and evenings.

4. Imposition of mandatory civil money penalties for each instance of serious chronic violations.

5. Emphasis on facilities owned by corporate chains that have a history of noncompliance.

6. Additional training for surveyors in states that HCFA believes are not protecting residents adequately and increased federal review of state inspections.

7. Increased scrutiny of nursing homes' ability to prevent bedsores, dehydration, and malnutrition.

8. State inspectors will review each nursing home's systems for the prevention of resident abuse, misappropriation, and neglect; facilities will be required to share the plan of these systems with residents and their families.

9. States that are found to perform surveys unsatisfactorily could lose the federal funding that supports survey activity and HCFA would instead contract with another entity for the survey function.

10. HCFA would work with law enforcement agencies to ensure that state survey agencies refer cases for prosecution under federal civil and criminal laws, especially in cases involving harm to residents.

11. Finally, the survey results and violation (citation) histories of nursing homes would be posted on the Internet.

Each of these steps has value, but a critical weakness remains: the survey process will never provide ongoing oversight, advocacy, and interaction at the individual resident level. Inspections, incentives, and accreditation all seek to define quality from the perspectives of regulators, providers, and payer sources. But it is the informed, empowered consumer and family member or decision maker who can advocate for quality at the individual level each and every day.

Informed and empowered resident councils and committees, family councils, and support groups can raise issues on a facilitywide basis, with a unified voice that is difficult not to hear. Informed and empowered advocacy groups and local aging units can become players in keeping quality-of-care and quality-of-life issues at the top of facility agendas in their community.

With all the emphasis placed on quality by compulsion through the threat of sanctions and all the reportorial hyperbole at each instance of poor care and abuse, it is easy to forget that most people who use nursing home care experience good quality of care and quality of life. Most facilities meet and often exceed what federal and state standards mandate. Many facilities are finding innovative ways to work and creative ways to enhance the living environment for their residents, and there are groups and individuals spurring on such change.

For example, Dr. William Thomas, creator of the "Eden Alternative," advocates fresh thinking on how nursing homes behave. The Eden Alternative advocates eliminating loneliness, helplessness, and boredom, which can become major afflictions for elders in nursing homes, by keeping the environment enlivened with plants, animals, and children and engaging residents in spontaneous, meaningful activities including caregiving. To learn more about the Eden Alternative:

> The Eden Alternative
> 742 Turnpike Road
> Sherburne, NY 13460
> phone: (607) 674-5232
> fax: (607) 674-6723
> e-mail: eden@norwich.net
> Internet:http://www.edenalt.com

The National Citizens' Coalition for Nursing Home Reform (NCCNHR) has continued to work for the betterment of nursing homes nationwide. The coalition is a cooperative effort of the National Institute on Aging and the Administration on Aging. It works to provide information to consumers, to foster citizen groups and ombudsman programs, and to promote improvements in the delivery of care and improvements in public policy. NCCNHR can be reached at

> National Citizens' Coalition for Nursing Home Reform
> 1424 16th Street, NW
> Suite 202
> Washington, DC 20036-2211
> phone: (202) 332-2275
> fax: (202) 332-2949
> Internet:http://www.aoa.dhhs.gov/aoa/dir/144.html

The fact that thousands of dedicated, skilled people work literally day and night to make nursing homes excellent in every way should not be lost. Their shortcomings are frequently overstated; the caregivers who are devoted to their profession are frequently denigrated, and their incredible skill levels depreciated. Those in the care of such devoted professionals generally experience good care and enjoy quality of life.

There are a growing number of alternatives to nursing home care, and that's encouraging. Still, there are going to be thousands of individuals each year who require nursing home care, if only for a relatively short time. For those individuals, there should be the assurance that life, even in a nursing home, can and should be rich, fulfilling, and safe. The nursing home *can* be a place with music, laughter, dancing, friends, family, and warmth. It can be a source of support, comfort, and solace. It is also a place of recovery and renewal of physical health and restoration to independence.

The role of consumers and families in shaping the delivery of long-term care is crucial. This book can replace confusion, guilt, and fear with empowerment, control, and advocacy at the individual level. It is necessary for consumers and family members to speak knowledgeably and forcefully to ensure that those responsible for nursing home care hear their voice.

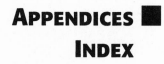

APPENDICES

INDEX

COMMON HEALTH CARE ACRONYMS AND ABBREVIATIONS

This listing of acronyms and abbreviations is intended to help consumers interpret the medical record and navigate through health care–related documents and forms. It is intended to allow consumers to examine medical records with a greater degree of understanding. This listing will enable consumers to know the meaning of an acronym or abbreviation, but not necessarily what it means in the context of an individual case. The intent is to facilitate questions that are clear and on target when participating in care planning and evaluation of quality of care. Care should be taken not to jump to conclusions or to attempt self-diagnosis based on fragments of the medical record.

AAAHC   Accreditation Association for Ambulatory Health Care

AAHA   American Association of Homes for the Aging

A&O × 1, 2, or 3   Alert and oriented times one (to person), two (person and place), or three (person, place, and time)

AARP   American Association of Retired Persons

abd   abdomen

ABG   arterial blood gas

ABMS   American Board of Medical Specialists

ABMT   autologous bone marrow transplant

ac   *ante cibos,* before meals

ACLS   advanced cardiac life support

ACTH   adrenocorticotrophic hormone

ADA   American Dietetic Association

ADC   Alzheimer Disease Center

ADEAR Alzheimer's Disease Education and Referral Center

ADH antidiuretic hormone

ADL activities of daily living

ad lib *ad libitum,* as desired

ADN associate degree–nursing

AFB acid-fast bacillus

AHA American Heart Association or American Hospital Association

AHCPR Agency for Health Care Policy and Research

AIDS acquired immunodeficiency syndrome

AKA above the knee amputation

AM morning

AMA American Medical Association

AMI acute myocardial infarction (heart attack)

amt amount

ap apical pulse

APN advanced practice nurse

ARC AIDS-related complex

ARDS adult respiratory distress syndrome

AROM active range of motion

ASA acetylsalisylic acid (aspirin)

ASCVD atherosclerotic cardiovascular disease

ASHD arteriosclerotic heart disease

ATLS advanced trauma life support

ax axillary or axis

B&B bowel and bladder

BG blood glucose

bid *bis in die,* twice a day

BKA below the knee amputation

BLS basic life support

BM bowel movement

BMR basal metabolic rate

BP blood pressure

BPH benign prostatic hypertrophy/hyperplasia

bpm beats per minute

BQC, BQA Bureau of Quality Compliance or Assurance

BRP bathroom privileges

BS bachelor of science, blood sugar, or bowel sounds

BSN bachelor of science–nursing

bta bilaterally to auscultation

BUN blood urea nitrogen

c, c̄ *cum,* with

CA cancer, carcinoma, cardiac arrest

CABG coronary artery bypass graft

CAD coronary artery disease

C&S culture and sensitivity

cath catheter

CBC complete blood count

CBD continuous bladder drainage

CBR complete bed rest

cc cubic centimeter

CDC Centers for Disease Control

CHD coronary heart disease

CHF congestive heart failure

CMS circulation, motion, and sensation

CNA certified nursing assistant

CNS central nervous system

c/o complains of

COBRA Consolidated Omnibus Budget Reconciliation Act

COLD chronic obstructive lung disease

CON certificate of need

COPD chronic obstructive pulmonary disease

CORF comprehensive outpatient rehabilitation facility

COTA certified occupational therapy assistant

CP chest pain

CPR cardiopulmonary resuscitation

CQI continuous quality improvement

CRNA certified registered nurse anesthetist

CSF cerebrospinal fluid

CV cardiovascular

CVA cerebrovascular accident (stroke)

CVR cardiovascular respiratory

CVU clean voided urine

d day

D&I dry and intact

DC or D/C discontinue

DHHS Department of Health and Human Services

DJD degenerative joint disease

DM diabetes mellitus

DME durable medical equipment

DMERC durable medical equipment regional carrier

DNR do not resuscitate

DOA dead on arrival

DON director of nursing

DRG diagnosis-related group

drsng, drsg dressing

DSS Department of Social Services

dss ducosate sodium (laxative; e.g., Colace)

Dx diagnosis

ea each

ECF extended care facility, or extracellular fluid

ECG, EKG electrocardiogram

ECT   electroconvulsive therapy

ED   emergency department

EEG   electroencephalogram

EMG   electromyogram

EMS   emergency medical services

EMT   emergency medical technician

EN   enteral nutrition

ENT   ear, nose, and throat

EOB   explanation of benefits

ER   emergency room

ERCP   endoscopic retrograde cholangiopancreatography

ERISA   Employee Retirement Income Security Act

ERT   estrogen replacement therapy

ESR   erythrocyte sedimentation rate (lab value)

ET   endotracheal

ETOH   ethyl alcohol

F   Fahrenheit

f, Fe   female

FB   foreign body

FBS   fasting blood sugar

FDA   Food and Drug Administration

FEHBP   Federal Employees Health Benefit Program

flu vax   influenza vaccine

FQHMO   federally qualified health maintenance organization

Fr   French (catheter size designation)

f/r   full and regular pulse

ft   foot or feet

f/u   follow-up

FUO   fever of unknown origin

fwb   full weight bearing

Fx   fracture

g   gram(s)

GERD   gastroesophageal reflux disease

GFR   glomerular filtration rate

GI   gastrointestinal

gr   grain(s)

gt   drop

gtt   *guttae,* drops

G-tube   gastrostomy tube

GU   genitourinary

GYN   gynecology or gynecological

h   hour(s)

h/a   headache

H&H   hemoglobin and hematocrit

H&P   history and physical

HBIg   hepatitis B immunoglobulin

HBV   hepatitis B virus

HCFA   Health Care Financing Administration

HCPCS   HCFA Common Procedural Coding System

Hct   hematocrit (blood lab value)

HCTZ   hydrochlorothiazide (a diuretic and antihypertensive medication)

HCVD   hypertensive cardiovascular disease

HEDIS®   Health Plan Employer Data and Information Set

Hgb   hemoglobin (blood lab value)

HIV   human immunodeficiency virus

HMO   health maintenance organization

H/O   history of

HOB   head of bed

HOH   hard of hearing

HPI   history of present illness

hs   *hora somni,* hour of sleep or "at bedtime"

HTN   hypertension

Hx   history

I&O   intake and output (of fluids)

ICD-9   *International Classification of Diseases,* 9th edition

ICS   intercostal space (between the ribs)

ICU   intensive care unit

ID   identification

IDDM   insulin-dependent diabetes mellitus

Ig   immunoglobulin

IH   infectious hepatitis

IM   intramuscular (injection)

inc   incontinent

inf   infection or inferior

INH   isoniazid (isonicotinic acid hydrazide, antitubercular medication)

inj   injection or injectable

integ   integument (skin)

IPO   insured product option

IPPB   intermittent positive-pressure breathing

I/S   instruct/supervise

IV   intravenous

IVP   intravenous pyelogram

IVPB   intravenous piggyback

JCAHO   Joint Commission on Accreditation of Healthcare Organizations

JVD   jugular venous distention

KCL, K+   potassium chloride

kg   kilogram(s)

KS   Kaposi's sarcoma

KUB   kidney, ureter, and bladder (usually refers to X-rays)

(L) or lt   left

l   liter (1,000 cc or ml)

lap   laparotomy

lb   pound(s)

LBP   low back pain

LE   lower extremities

LLE   left lower extremity

LLQ   left lower quadrant

l/min   liters per minute

LOC   level of consciousness or loss of consciousness

LOS   length of stay

LPN   licensed practical nurse

LTC   long-term care

LUE   left upper extremity

LUQ   left upper quadrant

LVN   licensed vocational nurse

m   meter(s) or minim

MA   master of arts, Medicaid, or mental age

MAR   medication administration record

max   maximum

mcg   microgram(s)

MCO   managed care organization

MD   medical doctor

med   medication

mEq   milliequivalent(s)

mg   milligram(s)

MHU   mental health unit

MI   myocardial infarction (also AMI or heart attack)

MICU   medical intensive care unit

min   minute(s)

ml   milliliter(s) (1,000 ml = 1 l)

mm   millimeter(s) (1,000 mm = 1 m)

mmol   millimole(s)

mod   moderate

mol   mole

MOM   milk of magnesia

MPPPA   Medicaid Prudent Pharmaceutical Purchasing Act of 1990

MR   mental retardation

MRI   magnetic resonance imaging

MRSA   methycillin-resistant staph aureus

MS   master of science, morphine sulfate, or multiple sclerosis

MSO   management services organization

MSS   medical social services

MSW   master of social work or medical social worker

NAIC   National Association of Insurance Commissioners

NANDA North American Nursing Diagnosis Association

N&V nausea and vomiting

NAS no added salt

NC nasal cannula

NCCNHR National Citizens' Coalition for Nursing Home Reform

NCI National Cancer Institute

NCQA National Committee for Quality Assurance

NDC National Drug Code

NF National Formulary

NG nasogastric

NIDDM non–insulin-dependent diabetes mellitus

NIH National Institutes of Health

NIMH National Institute of Mental Health

NKA no known allergy

NKDA no known drug allergy

NLN National League for Nursing

no number

noc nocturnal, at night

non-par nonparticipating provider

NP nurse practitioner

NPDB National Practitioner Data Bank

NPO *nil per os,* nothing by mouth

NS normal saline or not significant

NSAID nonsteroidal anti-inflammatory drug

NSR normal sinus rhythm

NTG nitroglycerin

NWB non–weight bearing

o oral

OBRA Omnibus Budget Reconciliation Act

OCI Office of the Commissioner of Insurance

OD *oculus dexter,* right eye

OHD organic heart disease

OIG Office of the Inspector General

OMB Office of Management and Budget

OOP out of plan or out of pocket

OPHC Office of Prepaid Health Care

OPT outpatient physical therapy

OR operating room

O/R observe and report

OS *oculus sinister,* left eye

os *os,* mouth

OT occupational therapist

OTA Office of Technology Assessment

OTC over the counter (nonprescription drug)

O₂ oxygen

OU *oculus uterque,* each eye

oz ounce(s)

P pulse

p *post,* after

PA or PA-C physician's assistant

PAC premature atrial contraction

P&A percussion and auscultation

par participating provider

pc *post cibos,* after meals

PCA patient-controlled analgesia

PCN penicillin

PCP primary care physician

P/E physical examination

PEEP positive end-expiratory pressure

PERRLA pupils equal, round, reactive to light and accommodation

pH potential (concentration) of hydrogen (measure of the acidity of a substance)

PHO physician–hospital organization

PJC premature junctional contraction

PKU phenylketonuria

PM evening

po *per os,* by mouth

POMR problem-oriented medical record

POS point of service

pos position

PO$_2$ partial pressure of oxygen

p/p pathophysiology

ppm parts per million

PPO preferred provider organization

PPS prospective pricing system

PRN *pro re nata,* as needed

PRO peer review organization

PROM passive range of motion

psi pounds per square inch

PSO provider-sponsored organization

PSRO professional standards review organization

PT physical therapy or therapist

PT or Pro-time prothrombin time (blood lab value)

pt pint(s)

Pt patient

PTCA percutaneous transluminal coronary angioplasty

PTT partial thromboplasin time (blood lab value)

PUD peptic ulcer disease

PVC premature ventricular contraction

PVD peripheral vascular disease

PVP-iodine povidone (polyvinylpyrrolidone) iodine

PVR   postvoid residual

PWB   partial weight bearing

Px   past history or physical examination

PZI   protamine zinc insulin

q   *quodque*, every or each

q2h   *quaque secunda hora*, every two hours

QA   quality assurance

QAAC   Quality Assessment and Assurance Committee

qAM   every (*quaque*) morning

qd   *quaque die*, every day

QI   quality improvement or qualified individual (Medicare)

qid   *quater in die*, four times a day

QIO   quality improvement organization

QMB   qualified Medicare beneficiary

qod   every other day (from qad, *quoque alternis die*)

qs   *quantum sufficiat*, a sufficient quantity

qt   quart(s)

R   respiration

RQ   respiratory quotient

RA   rheumatoid arthritis

RAI   Resident Assessment Instrument

RAP   Resident Assessment Protocol

RBBB   right bundle-branch block (type of conduction defect in the heart)

RBC   red blood cell

ref   refused

res   resident

RF   renal failure or respiratory failure

RIND   reversible ischemic neural deficit

RLE   right lower extremity

RLQ   right lower quadrant

RN   registered nurse

r/o   rule out

ROM   range of motion

RT   respiratory therapist or therapy

rt   right

RUE   right upper extremity

RUQ   right upper quadrant

RVF   right ventricular failure

RVR   rapid ventricular response

Rx   prescription

S   signa (in prescriptions referring to patient instructions given)

s or s̄   *sine*, without

S$_1$, S$_2$ first and second heart sounds

S$_3$ ventricular heart sound

S₄ atrial heart sound

SA sinoatrial

SAD seasonal affective disorder

sat. saturation

SCU specialized care unit

SGOT serum glutamic-oxaloacetic transaminase (blood lab value)

SGPT serum glutamic-pyruvic transaminase

SH serum hepatitis

SI Système Internationale (international system of units of measure)

SICU surgical intensive care unit

sl sublingual

SLE systemic lupus erythematosus

SLMB specified low-income Medicare beneficiary

SLP speech language pathologist

SN skilled nursing or student nurse

SNF skilled nursing facility

SOAP charting method: subjective, objective, assessment, plan

sol or soln solution

s/p status post (after an event or procedure)

SQ or sub-q subcutaneous

SS sterile solution, soap suds

s/s signs and symptoms

SSE soap suds enema

ST speech therapist or therapy

STD sexually transmitted disease

STP standard temperature and pressure

supp suppository

suppl supplement

SVT supraventricular tachycardia

Sx symptoms

T temperature

tab tablet

TB tuberculosis

tbs tablespoon(s)

TENS transcutaneous electrical nerve stimulation

TIA transient ischemic attack

tid *ter in die,* three times a day

TKO to keep open (referring to an IV flow rate)

TMJ temporomandibular joint

tol tolerated

TPA tissue plasminogen activator

TPN total parenteral nutrition

TPR temperature, pulse, respiration

TQM total quality management

tsp teaspoon(s)

TURB-T transurethral resection of the bladder-tumor

TURP transurethral resection of the prostate

Tx treatment

u/a urinalysis

UAO upper airway obstruction

UE upper extremities

UGI upper gastrointestinal tract X-ray

UM utilization management

UR utilization review

URI upper respiratory infection

USP United States Pharmacopeia

USPHS United States Public Health Service

UTI urinary tract infection

v vein

V visual or volt

VA Veterans Administration

VF ventricular fibrillation

VH viral hepatitis

VLDL very low density lipoprotein

VS vital signs

VSS vital signs stable

VT or V-tach ventricular tachycardia

W watt

wa while awake

WB weight bearing

WBC white blood cell

WBQC wide-base quad cane

w/c wheelchair

wcb wheelchair bound

WNL within normal limits

wt weight

x times

STATE MEDICAID OFFICES

Alabama
800-362-1504

Alaska
800-770-5650

American Samoa
011-684-633-4590

Arizona
602-417-4680

Arkansas
501-682-8487

California
800-952-5253

Colorado
303-866-2993

Connecticut
860-424-5008

Delaware
302-577-4901

District of Columbia
202-727-0735 or 202-724-5506

Florida
850-488-3560

Georgia
800-282-4536

Guam
011-671-734-7264

Hawaii
808-586-5391

Idaho
208-334-5747

Illinois
800-252-8635

Indiana
317-232-4966

Iowa
515-281-8621

Kansas
785-296-3349

Kentucky
502-564-6884

Louisiana
504-342-3855 or 504-342-5716

Maine
207-624-5277

Maryland
410-767-1432

Massachusetts
800-841-2900

Michigan
800-642-3195

Minnesota
800-657-3739

Mississippi
601-359-6056

Missouri
573-751-3425

Montana
406-444-5900

Nebraska
402-471-9147

Nevada
702-687-4775

New Hampshire
603-271-4344

New Jersey
609-588-2600

New Mexico
505-827-3100

New York
518-486-4803

North Carolina
800-662-7030

North Dakota
800-755-2604

Northern Mariana Islands
011-670-234-8950, ext. 2905

Ohio
800-324-8680

Oklahoma
405-530-3439

Oregon
503-945-5811

Pennsylvania
717-787-1870

Puerto Rico
787-765-1230

Rhode Island
404-464-2121

South Carolina
803-253-6100

South Dakota
605-773-3495

Tennessee
615-741-0213

Texas
512-438-3219

U.S. Virgin Islands
809-774-4624

Utah
801-538-6155

Vermont
802-241-2880

Virginia
804-786-7933

Washington
800-562-3022

West Virginia
800-642-3607

Wisconsin
608-266-2522

Wyoming
307-777-5500

State Health Insurance Information and Counseling Phone Numbers

Free assistance is available for people with questions on Medicare, Medicaid, Medigap private and long-term care insurance, and other health insurance-related questions. The 800 numbers apply only to in-state calls. For additional assistance, call the Medicare Hot Line: 1-800-638-6833.

Alabama
800-243-5463

Alaska
800-478-6065

Arizona
800-432-4040

Arkansas
800-852-5494

California
800-927-4357

Colorado
303-894-7499, ext 356

Connecticut
800-443-9946

Delaware
800-336-9500

District of Columbia
202-676-3900

Florida
904-922-2073

Georgia
800-669-8387

Hawaii
808-586-0100

Idaho
800-247-4422

Illinois
800-548-9034

Indiana
800-452-4800

Iowa
515-281-5705

Kansas
800-432-3535

Kentucky
800-372-2973

Louisiana
800-259-5301

Maine
800-750-5353

Maryland
800-243-3425

Massachusetts
800-882-2003

Michigan
517-373-8230

Minnesota
800-882-6262

Mississippi
800-948-3090

Missouri
800-390-3330

Montana
800-332-2272

Nebraska
402-471-4506

Nevada
800-307-4444

New Hampshire
603-271-4642

New Jersey
800-792-8820

New Mexico
800-432-2080

New York
800-333-4114

North Carolina
800-443-9354

North Dakota
800-247-0560

Ohio
800-686-1578

Oklahoma
405-521-6628

Oregon
800-722-4134

Pennsylvania
717-783-8975

Puerto Rico
809-721-5710

Rhode Island
800-322-2880

South Carolina
800-868-9095

South Dakota
605-773-3656

Tennessee
800-525-2816

Texas
800-252-3439

U.S. Virgin Islands
809-774-2991

Utah
801-538-3910

Vermont
800-642-5119

Virginia
800-552-3402

Washington
800-397-4422

West Virginia
304-558-3317

Wisconsin
800-242-1060

Wyoming
800-438-5768

PART B MEDICARE CARRIERS

Phone the relevant number below for questions or problems with Medicare Part B benefits.

Alabama   Blue Cross Blue Shield of Alabama
800-292-8855 or 205-988-2244

Alaska   Blue Cross Blue Shield of North Dakota
800-444-4606

American Samoa   Blue Cross Blue Shield of North Dakota
800-444-4606

Arizona   Blue Cross Blue Shield of North Dakota
800-444-4606

Arkansas   Arkansas Blue Cross Blue Shield
800-482-5525 or 501-378-2320

California   Transamerica Occidental Life Insurance
800-675-2266 or 213-748-2311

Colorado   Blue Cross Blue Shield of North Dakota
800-444-4606

Connecticut   United Health Care
800-982-6819 (in-state) or 203-237-8592

Delaware   Medicare Customer Service Center
800-444-4606

District of Columbia   Medicare Customer Service Center
800-444-4606

From *Medicare and You,* from the Health Care Financing Administration.

Florida   Blue Cross Blue Shield of Florida
800-333-7586

Georgia   Cahaba
800-727-0827 or 912-927-0934

Guam   Blue Cross Blue Shield of North Dakota
800-444-4606

Hawaii   Blue Cross Blue Shield of North Dakota
800-444-4606

Idaho   CIGNA Medicare
800-627-2782 or 615-244-5650

Illinois   Wisconsin Physician's Service
800-642-6930 or 312-938-8000; TDD 800-535-6152

Indiana   AdminiStar Federal
800-622-4792 or 317-842-4152

Iowa   Blue Cross Blue Shield of North Dakota
515-245-4785 or 800-532-1285

Kansas   Blue Cross Blue Shield of Kansas
800-432-3531 (in-state) or 800-432-0216

Kentucky   AdminaStar Federal
800-999-7608 or 502-425-6759

Louisiana   Arkansas Blue Cross Blue Shield
800-462-9666 or 504-927-3490

Maine   National Heritage Insurance Company
800-492-0919 or 781-741-5256

Maryland   Medicare Customer Service Center
800-444-4606

Massachusetts   National Heritage Insurance Company
800-882-1228 or 781-741-5256

Michigan   Wisconsin Physician's Service
800-482-4045

Minnesota   United Health Care
800-352-2762 or 612-884-7171

Mississippi   United Health Care
800-682-5417 or 601-956-0372

Missouri   Blue Cross Blue Shield of Kansas
816-561-0900 or 800-392-3070 or 314-843-8880

Montana   Blue Cross Blue Shield of Montana
800-332-6146 or 406-444-8350

Nebraska   Blue Cross Blue Shield of Kansas
800-633-1113

Nevada   Blue Cross Blue Shield of North Dakota
800-444-4606

New Hampshire   National Heritage Insurance Company
800-447-1142 or 781-741-5256

New Jersey   Xact Medicare Service
800-462-9306

New Mexico   Arkansas Blue Cross Blue Shield
800-423-2925 or 505-872-2551

New York   Empire Blue Cross/Blue Shield
800-442-8430 (Bronx, Brooklyn, Columbia, Delaware, Dutchess, Greene, Manhattan, Nassau, Orange, Putnam, Richmond, Rockland, Suffolk, Sullivan, Ulster, and Westchester)

Group Health Insurance, Queens
718-721-1770

BC/BS of Western New York
800-252-6550

North Carolina   CIGNA
800-672-3071 or 336-665-0348

North Dakota   Blue Shield of North Dakota
800-332-6681 or 800-247-2267 or 701-277-2363

Northern Mariana Islands   Blue Cross Blue Shield of
North Dakota
800-444-4606

Ohio   Nationwide Mutual Insurance Co.
800-282-0530

Oklahoma   Arkansas Blue Cross Blue Shield
800-522-9079 or 405-848-7711

Oregon   Blue Cross Blue Shield of North Dakota
800-444-4606

Pennsylvania   Xact Medicare Service
800-382-1274

Puerto Rico   Triple S, Inc.
800-981-7015 or 787-749-4900 (metro areas)

Rhode Island   Blue Cross Blue Shield of Rhode Island
800-662-5170 or 401-861-2273

South Carolina   Blue Cross Blue Shield of South Carolina
800-868-2522 or 803-788-3882

South Dakota   Blue Cross Blue Shield of North Dakota
800-437-4762

Tennessee   CIGNA Medicare
800-342-8900 or 615-244-5650

Texas   Blue Cross Blue Shield of Texas
800-442-2620

U.S. Virgin Islands   Triple S, Inc.
800-474-7448

Utah   Blue Cross Blue Shield of Utah
800-426-3477

Vermont   National Heritage Insurance Company
800-447-1142 or 781-741-5256

Virginia   Medicare Customer Service Center
800-444-4606 (Arlington and Fairfax counties)

United HealthCare
800-552-3423 (remainder of state)

Washington   Blue Cross Blue Shield of North Dakota
800-444-4606

West Virginia   Nationwide Mutual Insurance Co.
800-848-0106 or 614-249-7137

Wisconsin   Medicare WPS
800-944-0051 or 608-221-3330; TTY/TDD: 800-828-2837

Wyoming   Blue Cross Blue Shield of North Dakota
800-442-2371 or 307-632-9381

Medicare Durable Medical Equipment Regional Carriers

To discuss bills or Medicare coverage on medical equipment, call the numbers below.

Alabama, Arkansas, Colorado, Florida, Georgia, Kentucky, Louisiana, Mississippi, New Mexico, North Carolina, Oklahoma, Puerto Rico, South Carolina, Tennessee, Texas, U.S. Virgin Islands   Palmetto Government Benefits Administrators Medicare DMERC Operations
800-213-5452; Spanish: 800-213-5446

Alaska, American Samoa, Arizona, California, Guam, Hawaii, Idaho, Iowa, Kansas, Missouri, Montana, Nebraska, Nevada, North Dakota, Northern Mariana Islands, Oregon, South Dakota, Utah, Washington, Wyoming   CIGNA Medicare
800-899-7095

Connecticut, Delaware, Maine, Massachusetts, New Hampshire, New Jersey, New York, Pennsylvania, Rhode Island, Vermont   United HealthCare
800-842-2050 or 717-735-7383

District of Columbia,* Illinois, Indiana, Maryland,* Michigan, Minnesota, Ohio, Virginia, West Virginia, Wisconsin   AdminiStar Federal, Inc.
800-270-2313 or *800-444-4606

Based on *Medicare and You,* from the Health Care Financing Administration.

MEDICARE PEER REVIEW ORGANIZATIONS

Phone the following numbers with complaints or questions dealing with quality of care.

Alabama   Alabama Quality Assurance Foundation
800-760-3540

Alaska   PRO-West
800-445-6941; TTY: 800-251-8890

American Samoa   Mountain Pacific Quality Health Foundation
800-524-6550 or 800-545-2550

Arizona   Health Service Advisory Group, Inc.
800-626-1577

Arkansas   Arkansas Foundation for Medical Care, Inc.
800-272-5528 or 501-649-8501

California   California Medical Review, Inc.
800-841-1602 or 415-882-5800

Colorado   Colorado Foundation for Medical Care
800-727-7086 or 303-695-3333

Connecticut   Connecticut Peer Review Organization, Inc.
800-553-7590 or 860-632-2008

Delaware   West Virginia Medical Institute, Inc.
800-642-8686, ext. 266 or 302-655-3077

District of Columbia   Delmarva Foundation for Medical Care, Inc.
800-999-3362

Based on *Medicare and You* from the Health Care Financing Administration.

Florida   Florida Medical Quality Assurance
800-844-0795 or 813-354-9111

Georgia   Georgia Medical Care Foundations
800-979-7217 or 404-982-7575

Guam   Mountain Pacific Quality Health Foundation
800-524-6550 or 800-545-2550

Hawaii   Mountain Pacific Quality Health Foundation
800-524-6550 or 800-545-2550

Idaho   PRO-West
800-445-6941 or 208-343-4617 (Boise);
TTY: 800-251-8890

Illinois   Illinois Foundation for Medical Care
800-647-8089

Indiana   HealthCare Excel
800-288-1499

Iowa   Iowa Foundation for Medical Care
800-752-7014 or 515-223-2900

Kansas   Kansas Foundation for Medical Care
800-432-0407 or 785-273-2552

Kentucky   HealthCare Excel
800-288-1499

Louisiana   Louisiana Health Care Review, Inc.
800-433-4958 or 504-926-6353

Maine   Northeast Health Care Quality Foundation
800-772-0151

Maryland   Delmarva Foundation for Medical Care
800-492-5811 or 800-645-0011 (outside Maryland)

Massachusetts   MassPRO
800-252-5533 or 781-890-0011

Michigan   Michigan Peer Review Organization
800-365-5899

Minnesota   Status Health
800-444-3423 or 612-854-3306

Mississippi   Mississippi Foundation for Medical Care
601-354-0304 or 800-844-0600

Missouri   Missouri Patient Care Review Foundation
800-347-1016

Montana   Mountain Pacific Quality Health Foundation
800-497-8232 or 406-443-4020

Nebraska   Iowa Foundation for Medical Care, the
Sunderbruch Corp.
800-247-3004 or 402-474-7471

Nevada   Health Insight
800-748-6773 or 702-385-9933 or 702-826-1996 (Reno)

New Hampshire   Northeast Health Care Quality
Foundation
800-772-0150 or 603-749-1641

New Jersey   The PRO of New Jersey, Inc.
800-624-4557 or 732-238-5570

New Mexico   New Mexico Medical Review Association,
Inc.
800-279-6824 or 505-998-9898

New York   Island Peer Review Organization, Inc.
800-331-7767 or 800-446-2247 (appeals)

North Carolina   Medical Review of North Carolina
919-851-2955 or 800-772-0468

North Dakota   North Dakota Health Care Review, Inc.
800-472-2902 or 701-852-4231

Northern Mariana Islands   Mountain Pacific Quality
Health Foundation
800-524-6550 or 808-545-2550

Ohio   Peer Review Systems, Inc.
800-837-0664 or 800-589-7337 (Ohio)

Oklahoma Oklahoma Foundation for Medical Quality
800-522-3414 or 405-840-2891

Oregon Oregon Medical Profession Review
800-344-4354 or 503-279-0100

Pennsylvania Keystone Peer Review Organization, Inc.
800-332-1914 or 717-564-8288

Puerto Rico Quality Improvement Professional Research
800-981-5062 or 787-753-6708

Rhode Island Rhode Island Quality Partners
800-662-5028

South Carolina Carolina Medical Review
800-922-3089 or 803-731-8225

South Dakota South Dakota Foundation for Medical Care
800-658-2285 or 605-336-3505

Tennessee Mid-South Foundation Care
800-489-4633

U.S. Virgin Islands Virgin Islands Medical Institute
809-778-6470

Utah Health Insight
800-274-2290 or 801-487-2290

Vermont Northeast Health Care Quality Foundation
603-749-1641 or 800-772-0151

Virginia Virginia Health Care Quality Central Review Organization (DC, MD, VA)
800-545-3814 or 804-289-5320 or 804-289-5397

Washington PRO-West
800-445-6941; TTY: 800-251-8890

West Virginia West Virginia Medical Institute, Inc.
800-642-8686, ext. 266 or 304-346-9864

Wisconsin Wisconsin Peer Review Organization (MetaStar)
800-362-2320 or 608-274-1940

Wyoming Mountain Pacific Quality Health Foundation
800-768-2572 (local) or 800-497-8232

STATE AGENCIES ON AGING

Alabama Alabama Commission on Aging, RSA Plaza, Suite 470, 770 Washington Avenue, Montgomery, AL 36130
334-242-5743; fax: 334-242-5594

Alaska Alaska Commission on Aging, Division of Senior Services, Department of Administration, Juneau, AK 99811-0209
907-465-3250; fax: 907-465-4716

American Samoa Territorial Administration on Aging, Government of American Samoa, Pago Pago, AS 96799
011-684-633-2207; fax: 011-684-633-2533

Arizona Aging and Adult Administration, Department of Economic Security, 1789 West Jefferson Street, 950A, Phoenix, AZ 85007
602-542-4446; fax: 602-542-6575

Arkansas Division Aging and Adult Services, Arkansas Department of Human Services, PO Box 1437, Slot 1412, 7th and Main Streets, Little Rock, AR 72201
501-682-2441; fax: 501-682-8155

California California Department of Aging, 1600 K Street, Sacramento, CA 95814
916-322-5290; fax: 916-324-1903

Colorado Aging and Adult Services, Department of Social Services, 110 16th Street, Suite 200, Denver, CO 80202-5202
303-620-4147; fax: 303-620-4189

Connecticut Division of Elderly Services, 25 Sigourney Street, 10th Floor, Hartford, CT 06106-5033
860-424-5277; fax: 860-424-4966

Delaware Delaware Division of Services for Aging and Adults with Physical Disabilities, Department of Health and Social Services, 1901 North DuPont Highway, New Castle, DE 19720
302-577-4791; fax: 302-577-4793

District of Columbia   District of Columbia Office on Aging, One Judiciary Square, 9th Floor, 441 Fourth Street, NW, Washington, DC 20001
202-724-5622; fax: 202-724-4979

Florida   Department of Elder Affairs, Building B, Suite 152, 4040 Esplanade Way, Tallahassee, FL 32399-7000
904-414-2000; fax: 904-414-2002

Georgia   Division of Aging Services, Department of Human Resources, 2 Peachtree Street NE, 18th Floor, Atlanta, GA 30303
404-657-5258; fax: 404-657-5285

Guam   Division of Senior Citizens, Department of Public Health and Social Services, PO Box 2816, Agana, Guam 96932
011-671-475-0263; fax: 671-477-2930

Hawaii   Hawaii Executive Office on Aging, 250 South Hotel Street, Suite 107, Honolulu, HI 96813
808-586-0100; fax: 808-586-0185

Idaho   Idaho Commission on Aging, 3380 Americana Terrace, Suite 120, Boise, ID 83706
208-334-3833; fax: 208-334-3033

Illinois   Illinois Department on Aging, 421 East Capitol Avenue, Suite 100, Springfield, IL 62701-1789
217-785-2870; fax: 217-785-4477

Chicago Office: 312-814-2630

Indiana   Bureau of Aging and In-Home Services, Division of Disability, Aging and Rehabilitative Services, Family and Social Services Administration, 402 West Washington Street, W454, PO Box 7083, Indianapolis, IN 46207-7083
317-232-7020; fax: 317-232-7867

Iowa   Iowa Department of Elder Affairs, Clemens Building, 3rd Floor, 200 Tenth Street, Des Moines, IA 50309-3609
515-281-5187; fax: 515-281-4036

Kansas   Department on Aging, New England Building, 503 South Kansas Avenue, Topeka, KS 66603-3404
785-296-4986; fax: 785-296-0256

Kentucky   Kentucky Division of Aging Services, Cabinet for Human Resources, 275 East Main Street, 6 West, Frankfort, KY 40621
502-564-6930; fax: 502-564-4595

Louisiana   Governor's Office of Elderly Affairs, PO Box 80374, 412 North 4th Street, 3rd Floor, Baton Rouge, LA 70802
504-342-7100; fax: 504-342-7133

Maine   Bureau of Elder and Adult Services, Department of Human Services, 35 Anthony Avenue, State House, Station 11, Augusta, ME 04333
207-626-5335; fax: 207-624-5361

Maryland   Maryland Office on Aging, State Office Building, Room 1007, 301 West Preston Street, Baltimore, MD 21201-2374
410-767-1100; fax: 410-333-7943

Massachusetts   Massachusetts Executive Office of Elder Affairs, One Ashburton Place, 5th Floor, Boston, MA 02108
617-727-7750; fax: 617-727-9368

Michigan   Office of Services to the Aging, PO Box 30026, Lansing, MI 48909-8176
517-373-8230; fax: 517-373-4092

Minnesota   Minnesota Board on Aging, 444 Lafayette Road, St. Paul, MN 55155-3843
612-296-2770; fax: 612-297-7855

Mississippi   Division of Aging and Adult Services, 750 State Street, Jackson, MS 39202
601-359-4925; fax: 601-359-4370

Missouri   Division on Aging, Department of Social Services, PO Box 1337, 615 Howerton Court, Jefferson City, MO 65102-1337
573-751-3082; fax: 573-751-8493

Montana   Senior and Long Term Care Division, Department of Public Health & Human Services, PO Box 8005, 48 North Last Chance Gulch, Helena, MT 59604
406-444-7788; fax: 406-444-7743

Nebraska   Department of Health and Human Services, Division on Aging, PO Box 95044, 301 Centennial Mall South, Lincoln, NE 68509-5044
402-471-2307; fax: 402-471-4619

Nevada   Nevada Division for Aging Services, Department of Human Resources, State Mail Room Complex, 340 North 11th Street, Suite 203, Las Vegas, NV 89101
702-486-3545; fax: 702-486-3572

New Hampshire   Division of Elderly and Adult Services, State Office Park South, 115 Pleasant Street, Annex Building 1, Concord, NH 03301-3843
603-271-4680; fax: 603-271-4643

New Jersey   Department of Health and Senior Services, Division of Senior Affairs, PO Box 807, Trenton, NJ 08625-0807
800-792-8820 or 609-588-3141; fax: 609-588-3601

New Mexico   State Agency on Aging, La Villa Rivera Building, 4th Floor, 224 East Palace Avenue, Santa Fe, NM 87501
505-827-7640; fax: 505-827-7649

New York   New York State Office for the Aging, 2 Empire State Plaza, Albany, NY 12223-1251
800-342-9871 or 518-474-5731; fax: 518-474-0608

North Carolina   Division of Aging, CB 29531, 693 Palmer Drive, Raleigh, NC 27626-0531
919-733-3983; fax: 919-733-0443

North Dakota   Department of Human Services, Aging Services Division, 600 South 2nd Street, Suite 1C, Bismarck, ND 58504
701-328-8910; fax: 701-328-8989

Northern Mariana Islands   CNMI Office on Aging, PO Box 2178, Commonwealth of the Northern Mariana Islands, Saipan, MP 96950
670-233-1320/1321; fax: 670-233-1327/0369

Ohio   Ohio Department of Aging, 50 West Broad Street, 9th Floor, Columbus, OH 43215-5928
614-466-5500; fax: 614-466-5741

Oklahoma   Services for the Aging, Department of Human Services, PO Box 25352, 312 Northeast 28th Street, Oklahoma City, OK 73125
405-521-2281/2327; fax: 405-521-2086

Oregon   Senior and Disabled Services Division, 500 Summer Street, Northeast, 2nd Floor, Salem, OR 97310-1015
503-945-5811; fax: 503-373-7823

Palau   State Agency on Aging, Republic of Palau, Koror, PW 96940
9-10-288-011-680-488-2736
fax: 9-10-288-680-488-1662/1597

Pennsylvania   Pennsylvania Department of Aging, Commonwealth of Pennsylvania, 555 Walnut Street, 5th Floor, Harrisburg, PA 17101-1919
717-783-1550; fax: 717-772-3382

Puerto Rico   Commonwealth of Puerto Rico, Governor's Office of Elderly Affairs, Call Box 50063, Old San Juan Station, San Juan, PR 00902
787-721-5710/4560/6121; fax: 787-721-6510

Rhode Island   Department of Elderly Affairs, 160 Pine Street, Providence, RI 02903-3708
401-277-2858; fax: 401-277-2130

South Carolina   Office on Aging, South Carolina Department of Health and Human Services, PO Box 8206, Columbia, SC 29201-8206
803-253-6177; fax: 803-253-4173

South Dakota   Office of Adult Services and Aging, Richard F. Kneip Building, 700 Governors Drive, Pierre, SD 57501-2291
605-773-3656; fax: 605-773-6834

Tennessee   Commission on Aging, Andrew Jackson Building, 9th Floor, 500 Deaderick Street, Nashville, TN 37243-0860
615-741-2056; fax: 615-741-3309

Texas   Texas Department on Aging, 4900 North Lamar, 4th Floor, Austin, TX 78751
512-424-6840; fax: 512-424-6890

U.S. Virgin Islands   Senior Citizen Affairs, Virgin Islands Department of Human Services, Knud Hansen Complex, Building A, 1303 Hospital Ground, Charlotte Amalie, VI 00802
809-774-0930; fax: 809-774-3466

Utah   Division of Aging and Adult Services, Box 45500, 120 North 200 West, Salt Lake City, UT 84145-0500
801-538-3910; fax: 801-538-4395

Vermont   Vermont Department of Aging and Disabilities, Waterbury Complex, 103 South Main Street, Waterbury, VT 05676
802-241-2400; fax: 802-241-2325

Virginia   Virginia Department for the Aging, 1600 Forest Avenue, Suite 102, Richmond, VA 23219-2327
804-662-9333; fax: 804-662-9354

Washington   Aging and Adult Services Administration, Department of Social and Health Services, PO Box 45050, Olympia, WA 98504-5050
360-586-8753; fax: 360-902-7848

West Virginia   West Virginia Bureau of Senior Services, Holly Grove, Building 10, 1900 Kanawha Boulevard East, Charleston, WV 25305-0160
304-558-3317; fax: 304-558-0004

Wisconsin   Bureau of Aging and Long Term Care Resources, Department of Health and Family Services, PO Box 7851, Madison, WI 53707
608-266-2536; fax: 608-267-3203

Wyoming   Office on Aging, Department of Health, 117 Hathaway Building, Room 139, Cheyenne, WY 82002-0480
307-777-7986; fax: 307-777-5340

ADDITIONAL RESOURCES

ACTION   Office of Public Affairs, 1100 Vermont Ave., NW, Washington, DC 20525
202-606-5108
ACTION is an independent federal agency which sponsors volunteer programs such as the Senior Companion Program, Retired Senior Volunteer Program (RSVP), the Foster Grandparent Program, and Volunteers in Service to America (VISTA).

Administration on Aging   330 Independence Ave., SW, Washington, DC 20201
202-619-1352
Eldercare Locator: 800-677-1116

Agency for Health Care Policy and Research (AHCPR)   Information and Publications Division, Executive Office Center, 2101 East Jefferson Street, Suite 501, Rockville, MD 20852
301-594-1368

Alzheimer's Association   919 North Michigan Avenue, Suite 1000, Chicago, IL 60611-1676
800-272-3900

Alzheimer's Disease Education and Referral Center (ADEAR)   PO Box 8250, Silver Spring, MD 20907-8250
800-438-4380

American Health Care Association   1201 L Street, NW, Washington, DC 20005
800-552-6843

Centers for Disease Control (CDC)   Office of Public Inquiries, 1600 Clifton Road, NE, Atlanta, GA 30333
404-639-3534

Commission on Civil Rights   1121 Vermont Avenue, NW, Washington, DC 20425
800-552-6843

Community Elder Care Awareness Campaigns Project Management and Coordination   Alzheimer's Association Public Policy Office, 1319 F. Street, NW, Suite 700, Washington, DC 20005
202-393-7737

Dementia Care and Respite Services Program Direction and Technical Assistance   Department of Psychiatry and Behavioral Medicine, Bowman Gray School of Medicine, Medical Center Boulevard, Winston-Salem, NC 27157-1087
919-716-4941

Department of Justice   Office of Public Affairs, Room 1216, 10th Street and Constitution Avenue, NW, Washington, DC 20530
202-514-2007
Project Safe Return—for cognitively impaired persons at risk for wandering away from home or health care settings.

Department of Veterans Affairs   810 Vermont Avenue, NW, Washington, DC 20420
202-233-3975
Check your local listings under "U.S. Government Dept. of Veterans Affairs" or Veterans Health Services and Research Administration.

Food and Drug Administration (FDA)   5600 Fishers Lane, Room 16-85, Rockville, MD 20857
301-443-3170

Health Care Financing Administration (HCFA)   6325 Security Boulevard, Baltimore, MD 21207
410-786-3000

National Elder Care Institute on Long-Term Care and Alzheimer's Disease   University of South Florida, Suncoast Gerontology Center, MDC Box 50, 12901 Bruce B. Downs Boulevard, Tampa, FL 33612
813-974-4355

National Health Information Center   PO Box 1133, Washington, DC 20013
800-336-4797

Second Surgical Opinion Program   Call Medicare Part B carrier in your area for phone numbers of physicians who provide second opinions in your area. See appendix D.

Social Security Administration
800-772-1213

U.S. Department of Health and Human Services   General phone number: 202-619-0257
AIDS Hot Line: 800-342-AIDS
Cancer Hot Line: 800-4-CANCER
Inspector General's Hotline: 800-HHS-TIPS; in Maryland: 800-838-3986
Hill-Burton free hospital care hot line: 800-638-0742; in Maryland: 800-492-0359

Veterans Benefits Administration   810 Vermont Avenue, NW, Washington, DC 20420
202-233-2567

STATE LONG-TERM CARE
FACILITY SURVEY AGENCIES

Alabama   Division of Licensure and Certification, Alabama Department of Public Health, 434 Monroe Street, PO Box 303017, Montgomery, AL 36130-3017
334-206-5100

Alaska   State of Alaska Department of Health and Social Services, Health Facilities Licensing and Certification, 4730 Business Park Boulevard, Suite 18, Building H, Anchorage, AK 99503-7137
907-561-8081

Arizona   Long-Term Care Program, Arizona Department of Health Services, 1647 East Morten Avenue, Suite 110, Phoenix, AZ 85020
602-255-1244

Arkansas   Office of Long-Term Care, Medical Services, Arkansas Department of Human Services, PO Box 8059, Slot 400, Little Rock, AR 72205
501-682-8486

California   Licensing and Certification Division, California Department of Health Services, PO Box 942732, 1800 Third Street, Suite 210, Sacramento, CA 94234-7320
916-445-4054

Colorado   Health Facilities Division, Building A, 2nd Floor, Colorado Department of Public Health and Environment, 4300 Cherry Creek Drive South, Room A5, Denver, CO 80222-1530
Office of the Executive Director: 303-692-2819

Connecticut   Division of Health Systems Regulation, Department of Public Health, 410 Capitol Avenue, MS 12HSR, Hartford, CT 06134-0308
860-509-7400

Delaware   Office of Health Facilities, Certification and Licensure, 3 Mill Road, Suite 308, Wilmington, DE 19806-2114
302-577-6666

District of Columbia   Service Facility Regulation Administration, Department of Consumer and Regulatory Affairs, PO Box 37200, Room 1007, 614 H Street, NW, 10th Floor, Washington, DC 20013-7200
202-727-7214

Florida   Division of Health Quality Assurance, Agency for Health Care Administration, 2727 Mahan Drive, Room 220, Talahassee, FL 32308-5403
904-487-2527

Georgia   Office of Regulatory Services, Georgia Department of Human Resources, 2 Peachtree Street, NW, 22nd Floor, Atlanta, GA 30303-3167
404-657-5700

Hawaii   Hospital and Medical Facilities Branch–Medicare Section, Hawaii State Department of Health, 1270 Queen Emma Street, Suite 1100, Honolulu, HI 96813-2307
808-586-4090

Idaho   Department of Health and Welfare, Bureau of Facility Standards, 450 West State Street, 3rd Floor, Boise, ID 83720-0036
208-334-6626

Illinois   Illinois Department of Public Health, 525 West Jefferson Street, 5th Floor, Springfield, IL 62761
217-782-2913

Indiana   Division of Long-Term Care, Indiana State Department of Health, 2 North Meridian Street, Section 4B, Indianapolis, IN 46204
317-233-7712

Iowa   Iowa Department of Inspection and Appeals, Health Facilities, Lucas State Office Building, 3rd Floor, Des Moines, IA 50319-0083
515-281-4233

Kansas   Kansas Bureau of Adult and Child Care Facilities, Kansas Department of Health and Environment, 900 Southwest Jackson Street, Suite 1001, Topeka, KS 66612-1290
913-296-1240

Kentucky   Division for Licensing and Regulation, Office of the Inspector General, Cabinet for Human Resources, Human Resources Building, 275 East Main Street, 4th Floor, Frankfort, KY 40621-0001
502-564-2800

Louisiana   Health Standards Section, Louisiana Department of Health and Hospitals, PO Box 3767, Baton Rouge, LA 70821-3767
504-342-0415

Maine   Maine Division of Licensing and Certification, 35 Anthony Avenue, 11 State House Station, Augusta, ME 04333-0011
207-624-5443

Maryland   Maryland Department of Health, Office of Health and Mental Hygiene, Metro Executive Center, 4th Floor, 4201 Patterson Avenue, Baltimore, MD 21215
410-764-2750

Massachusetts   Massachusetts Division of Health Care Quality, Department of Public Health, 10 West Street, 5th Floor, Boston, MA 02111
617-727-1299

Michigan   Michigan Department of Consumer and Industry Services, Division of Health Facility Licensing and Certification, 3423 North Martin Luther King Jr. Boulevard, PO Box 30664, Lansing, MI 48909
517-335-8449

Minnesota   Minnesota Department of Health, 717 Delaware Street, SE, PO Box 64900, St. Paul, MN 55164-0900
612-643-2171

Mississippi   Mississippi State Department of Health, Division of Certification and Licensure, PO Box 1700, Jackson, MS 39215-1700
601-354-7300

Missouri   Missouri Division of Aging
Missouri Department of Social Services, PO Box 1337, 615 Howerton Court, Jefferson City, MS 65102-1337
573-751-3082

Montana   Montana Department of Health and Human Services, Quality Assurance Division, Cogswell Building, PO Box 202951, Helena, MT 59620-2951
406-444-2037

Nebraska   Health Facility Licensure and Inspection, Nebraska Department of Health, PO Box 95007, Lincoln, NE 68509-5007
402-471-4961

Nevada   Bureau of Licensing and Certification/EMS, Nevada Department of Human Resources, 1550 East College Parkway, Suite 158, Carson City, NV 89710
702-687-4475

New Hampshire   New Hampshire Bureau of Health Facilities Administration, Division of Public Health Services, Licensing and Regulation Services, 6 Hazen Drive, Concord, NH 03301-6527
603-271-4592

New Jersey   Division of Health Facilities Evaluation and Licensing, New Jersey Department of Health, CN 367, Trenton, NJ 08625-0367
609-588-7733

New Mexico   Bureau of Health Facility Licensing and Certification, New Mexico Department of Health, 525 Camino de Los Marquez, Suite 2, Santa Fe, NM 87501
505-827-4200

New York   New York State Department of Health, Bureau of Long-Term Care Services, Corning Tower, Empire State Plaza, Room 1882, Albany, NY 12237
518-473-1564

North Carolina   North Carolina Division of Facility Services, Certification Section, 701 Barbour Drive, PO Box 29530, Raleigh, NC 27626-0530
919-733-7461

North Dakota   North Dakota Department of Health, Health Resources Section, 600 East Boulevard Avenue, Bismarck, ND 58505-2352
701-328-2352

Ohio   Ohio Department of Health, 246 North High Street, PO Box 118, Columbus, OH 43266-0118
614-752-9524

Oklahoma   Division of Long-Term Care, Oklahoma State Department of Health, 1000 Northeast 10th Street, Oklahoma City, OK 73117-1299
405-271-6868

Oregon   Oregon Health Division, Client Care Monitoring Unit, Health Care Licensure and Certification Section, 500 Summer Street, 2nd Floor, Salem, OR 97310-1015
503-945-6456 or 503-945-5833

Pennsylvania   Pennsylvania Department of Health, Division of Nursing Care Facilities, Room 526 Health and Welfare Building, Harrisburg, PA 17120
717-787-1816

Puerto Rico   Puerto Rico Department of Health, Former Ruiz Soler Hospital, Boyamon, PR 00959
809-781-1066

Puerto Rico and U.S. Virgin Islands   HCFA Region II, 26 Federal Plaza, Room 3811, New York, NY 10278
212-264-4680

Rhode Island   Rhode Island Division of Facilities Regulation, Department of Health, 3 Capitol Hill, Room 306, Providence, RI 02908-5097
401-222-2566

South Carolina   South Carolina Department of Health and Environmental Control, Bureau of Health Licensure and Certification, J. Marion Sims Building, 2600 Bull Street, Columbia, SC 29201-1708
803-737-7205

South Dakota   South Dakota Department of Health, Office of Health Care Facilities Licensure and Certification, 615 East 4th Street, Pierre, SD 57501-5070
605-773-3356

Tennessee   Tennessee Department of Health, Health Care Facilities, Cordell Hull Building, 1st Floor, 426 5th Avenue North, Nashville, TN 37247-0508
615-741-7539

Texas   Long-Term Care–Regulatory, Texas Department of Human Services, 1100 West 49th Street, Austin, TX 78756
512-834-6752

Utah   Utah Division of Health Systems Improvement, Long-Term Care Survey Section, PO Box 16990, Salt Lake City, UT 84114-2905
801-538-6559

Vermont   Vermont Division of Licensing and Protection, Ladd Hall, 103 South Main Street, Waterbury, VT 05671-2306
802-241-2345

Virginia   Virginia Department of Health, Office of Health Facilities Regulation, 3600 West Broad Street, Suite 216, Richmond, VA 23230
804-367-2102

Washington   Washington Department of Health, Aging and Adult Services Administration, Residential Care Services, PO Box 45600, Olympia, WA 98504-5600
360-493-2560

West Virginia   West Virginia Department of Health, Office of Health Facilities Licensure and Certification, 1900 Kanawha Boulevard East, Building 3, Suite 550, Charleston, WV 25305
304-558-0050

Wisconsin   Wisconsin Department of Health and Family Services, Bureau of Quality Assurance, 1 West Wilson Street, PO Box 309, Madison, WI 53701-0309
608-267-7157

Wyoming   Wyoming Department of Health, Office of Health Quality, First Bank Building, 8th Floor, 2020 Carey Avenue, Cheyenne, WY 82002-0480
307-777-7121

STATE LONG-TERM CARE
OMBUDSMAN OFFICES

State long-term care ombudsman programs investigate and resolve complaints made by or on behalf of residents of nursing homes, boards and care homes, and similar adult homes. The program also promotes policies and practices to improve the quality of life, health, safety, and rights of these residents.

Alabama State Long-Term Care Ombudsman, Commission on Aging, RSA Plaza, Suite 470, 770 Washington Avenue, Montgomery, AL 36130
334-242-5743; fax: 334-242-5594

Alaska State Long-Term Care Ombudsman, Older Alaskans Commission, 3601 C Street, Suite 260, Anchorage, AK 99503-5209
907-563-6393; fax: 907-561-3862

Arizona State Long-Term Care Ombudsman, Aging and Adult Administration, Department of Economic Security, 1789 West Jefferson, 950A, Phoenix, AZ 85007
602-542-6452; fax: 602-542-6575

Arkansas State Long-Term Care Ombudsman, Arkansas Division on Aging and Adult Services, 1417 Donaghey Plaza South, Slot 1412, Little Rock, AR 72203-1437
501-682-2441; fax: 501-682-8155

California State Long-Term Care Ombudsman, Department of Aging, 1600 K Street, Sacramento, CA 95814
916-322-5290; fax: 916-323-7299

Colorado State Long-Term Care Ombudsman, The Legal Center, 455 Sherman Street, Suite 130, Denver, CO 80203
303-722-0300; fax: 303-722-0720

Connecticut Acting State Long-Term Care Ombudsman, Elderly Services Division, 25 Sigourney Street, 10th Floor, Hartford, CT 06106-5033
860-424-5200; fax: 860-424-4966

Delaware State Long-Term Care Ombudsman, Delaware Services for Aging-Disabled, Oxford Building, Suite 200, 256 Chapman Road, Newark, DE 19702
302-453-3820 ext. 46; fax: 302-453-3836

District of Columbia   National Ombudsman Resource Center, c/o NCCNHR, 1424 16th Street, NW, Suite 202, Washington, DC 20036-2211
202-332-2275

Florida   State Long-Term Care Ombudsman, Florida State LTC Ombudsman Council, Holland Building, Room 270, 600 South Calhoun Street, Tallahassee, FL 32301
850-488-6190; fax: 850-488-5657

Georgia   State Long-Term Care Ombudsman, Division of Aging Services, 2 Peachtree Street NW, 18th Floor, Suite 18-129, Atlanta, GA 30303-3176
404-657-5319; fax: 404-657-5285

Hawaii   State Long-Term Care Ombudsman, Executive Office on Aging, Office of the Governor, 250 South Hotel St., Suite 107, Honolulu, HI 96813-2831
808-586-0100; fax: 808-586-0185

Idaho   State Long-Term Care Ombudsman, Office on Aging, PO Box 83720, 700 West Jefferson, Room 108, Boise, ID 83720-0007
208-334-3833; fax: 208-334-3033

Illinois   State Long-Term Care Ombudsman, Illinois Department on Aging, 421 East Capitol Avenue, Springfield, IL 62701-1789
217-785-3143; fax: 217-524-9644

Indiana   State Long-Term Care Ombudsman, Indiana Division of Aging and Rehabilitation Services, PO Box 7083-W454, 402 West Washington Street, W-454, Indianapolis, IN 46207-7083
317-232-7134; fax: 317-232-7867

Iowa   State Long-Term Care Ombudsman, Iowa Department of Elder Affairs, Clemens Building, 200 10th Street, 3rd Floor, Des Moines, IA 50309-3609
515-281-4656; fax: 515-281-4036

Kansas   Office of State Long-Term Care Ombudsman, 610 SW 10th Avenue, 2nd Floor, Topeka, KS 66612-1616
785-296-3017; fax: 785-296-3916

Kentucky   State Long-Term Care Ombudsman, Division of Aging Services, State LTC Ombudsman Office, 275 E Main Street, 5th Floor W, Frankfort, KY 40621
502-564-6930; fax: 502-564-4595

Louisiana   State Long-Term Care Ombudsman, Governor's Office of Elderly Affairs, State LTC Ombudsman Office, 412 North 4th Street, 3rd Floor, Baton Rouge, LA 70802
504-342-7100; fax: 504-342-7133

Maine   State Long-Term Care Ombudsman, 21 Bangor Street, PO Box 126, Augusta, ME 04332
207-621-1079; fax: 207-621-0509

Maryland   State Long-Term Care Ombudsman, Office on Aging, State Office Building, Room 1004, 301 West Preston Street, Baltimore, MD 21201
410-767-1091; fax: 410-333-7943

Massachusetts   State Long-Term Care Ombudsman, Executive Office of Elder Affairs, One Ashburton Place, 5th Floor, Boston, MA 02108-1518
617-727-7750

Michigan   State Long-Term Care Ombudsman, Citizens for Better Care, 416 North Homer Street, Station 101, Lansing, MI 48912-4700
517-886-6797; fax: 517-886-6349

Minnesota   State Long-Term Care Ombudsman, Office of Ombudsman for Older Minnesotans, 444 Lafayette Road, 4th Floor, St. Paul, MN 55155-3843
612-296-0382; fax: 612-297-5654

Mississippi   State Long-Term Care Ombudsman, Division of Aging and Adult Services, 750 North State Street, Jackson, MS 39202
601-359-4929; fax: 601-359-4970

Missouri   State Long-Term Care Ombudsman, Division on Aging, Department of Social Services, PO Box 1337, 615 Howerton Court, Jefferson City, MO 65102-1337
800-309-3282 or 573-526-0727; fax: 573-751-8687

Montana State Long-Term Care Ombudsman, Office on Aging, Department of Family Services, PO Box 8005, Helena, MT 59604-8005
406-444-4077; fax: 406-444-7743

Nebraska State Long-Term Care Ombudsman, Department on Aging, PO Box 95044, 301 Centennial Mall South, Lincoln, NE 68509-5044
402-471-2307; fax: 402-471-4619

Nevada State Long-Term Care Ombudsman, Division for Aging Services, Department of Human Resources, 340 North 11th Street, Suite 203, Las Vegas, NV 89101
702-486-3545; fax: 702-486-3572

New Hampshire State Long-Term Care Ombudsman, Health and Human Services, Office of the Ombudsman, 129 Pleasant Street, Concord, NH 03301-6505
603-271-4375; fax: 603-271-4771

New Jersey State Long-Term Care Ombudsman, 101 South Broad Street, CN808, 6th Floor, Trenton, NJ 08625-0808
609-588-3614; fax: 609-588-3365

New Mexico State Long-Term Care Ombudsman, State Agency on Aging, 228 East Palace Avenue, Suite A, Santa Fe, NM 87501
505-827-7640; fax: 505-827-7649

New York State Long-Term Care Ombudsman, Office for the Aging, 2 Empire State Plaza, Agency Building 2, Albany, NY 12223-0001
518-474-0108; fax: 518-474-7761

North Carolina State Long-Term Care Ombudsman, Division of Aging, CB 29531, 693 Palmer Drive, Raleigh, NC 27626-0531
919-733-3983; fax: 919-733-0443

North Dakota State Long-Term Care Ombudsman, Aging Services Division, Department of Human Services, 600 South 2nd Street, Suite 1C, Bismarck, ND 58504-5729
701-328-8915; fax: 701-328-8989

Ohio State Long-Term Care Ombudsman, Department of Aging, 50 West Broad Street, 9th Floor, Columbus, OH 43215-5928
614-644-7922; fax: 614-466-5741

Oklahoma State Long-Term Care Ombudsman, Aging Services Division, Department of Human Services, 312 Northeast, 28th Street, Suite 109, Oklahoma City, OK 73105
405-521-6734; fax: 405-521-2086

Oregon State Long-Term Care Ombudsman, Office of the LTC Ombudsman, 3855 Wolverine, NE, Suite 6, Salem, OR 97310
503-378-6533; fax: 503-373-0852

Pennsylvania State Long-Term Care Ombudsman, Department of Aging, 555 Walnut Street, 5th Floor, Forum Place, Harrisburg, PA 17101-1919
717-783-7247; fax: 717-772-3382

Puerto Rico State Long-Term Care Ombudsman, Governor's Office for Elder Affairs, Call Box 50063, Old San Juan Station, San Juan, Puerto Rico 00902
787-725-1515; fax: 787-721-6510

Rhode Island State Long-Term Care Ombudsman, Alliance for Better Long-Term Care, 422 Post Road, Suite 204, Warwick, RI 02888
401-785-3340; fax: 401-785-3391

South Carolina State Long-Term Care Ombudsman, Division on Aging, 202 Arbor Lake Drive, Suite 301, Columbia, SC 29223-4535
803-253-6177; fax: 803-253-4173

South Dakota State Long-Term Care Ombudsman, Office of Adult Services and Aging, 700 Governors Drive, Pierre, SD 57501-2291
605-773-3656; fax: 605-773-6834

Tennessee State Long-Term Care Ombudsman, Commission on Aging, Andrew Jackson Building, 9th Floor, 500 Deaderick Street, Nashville, TN 37243-0860
615-741-2056; fax: 615-741-3309

Texas State Long-Term Care Ombudsman, Department on Aging, PO Box 12786, Capitol Station, Austin, TX 78711
512-424-6875; fax: 512-424-6890

Utah State Long-Term Care Ombudsman, Division of Aging and Adult Services, Department of Social Services, PO Box 1367, Salt Lake City, UT 84103
801-538-3910; fax: 801-538-4395

Vermont State Long-Term Care Ombudsman, Vermont Legal Aid, Inc., 264 North Winooski, PO Box 1367, Burlington, VT 05402
802-863-5620; fax: 802-863-7152

Virginia State Long Term Care Ombudsman, Virginia Association of Area Agencies on Aging, 530 East Main Street, Suite 428, Richmond, VA 23219
804-644-2923; fax: 804-644-5640

Washington State Long-Term Care Ombudsman, Washington State Ombudsman Program, 1200 South 336th Street, Federal Way, WA 98003-7452
800-422-1384 or 253-838-6810; fax: 253-874-7831

West Virginia State Long-Term Care Ombudsman, Commission on Aging, 1900 Kanawha Boulevard East, Charleston, WV 25305-0160
304-558-3317; fax: 304-558-0004

Wisconsin State Long-Term Care Ombudsman, Board on Aging and Long-Term Care, 214 North Hamilton Street, Madison, WI 53703-2118
608-266-8945; fax: 608-261-6570

Wyoming State Long-Term Care Ombudsman, Wyoming Senior Citizens, Inc., PO Box 94, 953 Water Street, Wheatland, WY 82201
307-322-5553; fax: 307-322-3283

MEDICARE PART A FISCAL INTERMEDIARIES

To discuss questions on bills or coverage for hospital or skilled nursing home care, phone the numbers below.

Alabama   Blue Cross Blue Shield of Alabama
800-292-8855 or 205-988-2244

Alaska   Blue Cross Blue Shield of Washington and Alaska
425-670-1010

American Samoa   Hawaii Medical Service Association
808-948-5247

Arizona   Blue Cross of Arizona
602-864-4297

Arkansas   Arkansas Blue Cross Blue Shield
501-378-2000

California   Blue Cross of California
818-593-2006

Colorado   Blue Cross Blue Shield of Texas
903-463-4658

Connecticut   United Health Care
203-639-3222

Delaware   Empire Blue Cross and Blue Shield
800-444-4606

District of Columbia   Medicare Customer Service Center
800-444-4606

Florida   Blue Cross Blue Shield of Florida
904-355-8899

Based on *Medicare and You,* from the Health Care Financing Administration.

Georgia   Blue Cross Blue Shield of Georgia, Inc.
706-571-5371

Guam   Hawaii Medical Service Association
808-948-6247

Hawaii   Hawaii Medical Service Association
808-948-6247

Idaho   Medicare Northwest
503-721-7000

Illinois   Health Care Service Corporation
312-653-6266

Indiana   AdminiStar Federal
800-622-4792

Iowa   Wellmark, Inc.
712-279-8650

Kansas   Blue Cross Blue Shield of Kansas
800-445-7170

Kentucky   AdminaStar Federal
800-999-7608 or 502-425-6759

Louisiana   Blue Cross Blue Shield of Mississippi
601-936-0105 or 800-932-7644, ext. 4594

Maine   Associated Hospital of Maine
888-896-4997

Maryland   Medicare Customer Service Center
800-444-4606

Massachusetts   Associated Hospital of Maine
888-896-4997

Michigan   Health Care Service Corporation
800-482-4045 or 313-225-8317

Minnesota   Blue Cross Blue Shield of Minnesota
800-382-2000, ext. 5503 or 651-456-8000

Mississippi   United Health Care
800-682-5417 or 601-956-0372

Missouri   Blue Cross Blue Shield of Mississippi
800-932-7644

Montana   Blue Cross Blue Shield of Montana
800-447-7828 or 406-791-4086

Nebraska   Blue Cross Blue Shield of Nebraska
402-390-1850

Nevada   Blue Cross of California
818-593-2006

New Hampshire   New Hampshire–Vermont Health
Service
603-695-7204

New Jersey   Blue Cross Blue Shield of New Jersey
973-456-2112

New Mexico   Blue Cross Blue Shield of Texas
903-463-4658

New York   Empire Blue Cross/Blue Shield
800-442-8430

North Carolina   Blue Cross Blue Shield of North Carolina
919-688-5528

North Dakota   Blue Cross Blue Shield of North Dakota
800-332-6681 or 303-831-2661 (local)

Northern Mariana Islands   Hawaii Medical Service
Association
808-948-6247

Ohio   AdminiStar Federal
317-842-4151

Oklahoma   Group Health Services of Oklahoma (Blue
Cross Blue Shield of Oklahoma)
918-560-3367

Oregon   Medicare Northwest
503-721-7000

Pennsylvania   Veritus, Inc.
800-853-1419

Puerto Rico   Cooperative de Seguros de Vida Puerto Rico
787-758-9733

Rhode Island   Blue Cross Blue Shield of Rhode Island
401-861-2273 or 800-662-5170 (local)

South Carolina   Blue Cross Blue Shield of South Carolina
800-521-3761 or 803-432-5703 (local)

South Dakota   IASD Health Service Corp.
515-246-0126

Tennessee   Blue Cross Blue Shield of Tennessee
423-755-5955

Texas   Blue Cross Blue Shield of Utah
801-333-2410

U.S. Virgin Islands   Cooperative de Seguros de Vida
Puerto Rico
787-758-9733

Utah   Blue Cross Blue Shield of Utah
801-333-2410

Vermont   New Hampshire–Vermont Health Service
603-695-7200

Virginia   TRIGON Blue Cross Blue Shield
540-985-3931

Washington   Blue Cross Blue Shield of Washington and Alaska
425-670-1010

West Virginia   TRIGON Blue Cross Blue Shield
540-985-3931

Wisconsin   Blue Cross Blue Shield of Wisconsin
414-224-4954

Wyoming   Blue Cross Blue Shield of Wyoming
307-634-1393 or 800-442-2376

REGIONAL HOME HEALTH
INTERMEDIARIES

Contact these agencies for information about the Medicare Home Health and Hospice benefits.

Alabama, Arkansas, Florida, Georgia, Illinois, Indiana, Kentucky, Louisiana, Mississippi, New Mexico, North Carolina, Ohio, Oklahoma, South Carolina, Tennessee, Texas Palmetto Government Benefits Administrators
727-773-9225

Alaska, American Samoa, Arizona, California, Guam, Hawaii, Idaho, Nevada, Northern Mariana Islands, Oregon, Washington Blue Cross of California
818-593-2009

Colorado, Delaware, Iowa, Kansas, Missouri, Montana, Nebraska, North Dakota, Pennsylvania, South Dakota, Utah, Virginia, West Virginia, Wyoming Wellmark, Inc.
515-246-0126

District of Columbia, Maryland Medicare Customer Service Center
800-444-4606

Michigan, Minnesota, New Jersey, New York, Puerto Rico, U.S. Virgin Islands, Wisconsin Medicare Part A United Government Services
414-224-4954

Connecticut, Maine, Massachusetts, New Hampshire, Rhode Island, Vermont Associated Hospital Services of Maine
888-896-4997

Based on *Medicare and You*, from the Health Care Financing Administration.

STATE INSURANCE
DEPARTMENT OFFICES

Call the following numbers for information about Medicare supplemental insurance and long-term care insurance.

Alabama
334-269-3550

Alaska
907-269-7900

American Samoa
011-684-633-4116

Arizona
602-912-8444

Arkansas
800-852-5494

California
800-927-4357 or 213-897-8921

Colorado
800-930-3745

Connecticut
860-297-3800

Delaware
302-739-6266 or 800-336-9500

District of Columbia
202-727-0735 or 202-724-5506

Based on *Medicare and You,* from the Health Care Financing Administration.

Florida
850-488-3560

Georgia
800-282-4536

Guam
1-0-671-734-7264

Hawaii
808-586-5391

Idaho
208-334-5747

Illinois
800-252-8635

Indiana
317-232-4966

Iowa
515-281-8621

Kansas
785-296-3349

Kentucky
502-564-6885

Louisiana
504-342-3855/5716

Maine
207-624-5277

Maryland
410-767-1432

Massachusetts
800-841-2900

Michigan
800-642-3195

Minnesota
800-657-3739

Mississippi
601-359-6056

Missouri
573-751-3425

Montana
406-444-5900

Nebraska
402-471-9147

Nevada
702-687-4775

New Hampshire
603-271-4344

New Jersey
609-588-2600

New Mexico
505-827-3100

New York
518-486-4803

North Carolina
800-662-7030

North Dakota
800-755-2604

Northern Mariana Islands
011-670-234-8950, ext. 2905

Ohio
800-324-8680

Oklahoma
405-530-3439

Oregon
503-945-5811

Pennsylvania
717-787-1870

Puerto Rico
787-765-1230

Rhode Island
401-464-2121

South Carolina
803-253-6100

South Dakota
605-773-3495

Tennessee
615-741-0213

Texas
512-438-3219

U.S. Virgin Islands
809-774-4624

Utah
801-538-6155

Vermont
802-241-2880

Virginia
804-786-7933

Washington
800-562-3022

West Virginia
800-642-3607

Wisconsin
608-266-2522

Wyoming
307-777-5500

FEDERAL OFFICES OF CIVIL RIGHTS

Federal laws prohibit discrimination. Call these numbers for questions or possible discrimination complaints.

Connecticut, Maine, Massachusetts, New Hampshire, Rhode Island, Vermont
617-565-1340; TDD: 617-565-1343

New York, New Jersey, Puerto Rico, U.S. Virgin Islands
212-264-3313; TDD: 212-264-2355

Delaware, District of Columbia, Maryland, Pennsylvania, Virginia, West Virginia
215-861-4441; TDD: 215-861-4440

Alabama, Florida, Georgia, Kentucky, Mississippi, North Carolina, South Carolina, Tennessee
404-562-7886; TDD: 404-562-7884

Illinois, Indiana, Michigan, Minnesota, Ohio, Wisconsin
312-886-2359; TDD: 312-353-5693

Iowa, Kansas, Missouri, Nebraska
816-426-7277; TDD: 816-426-7065

Arkansas, Louisiana, New Mexico, Oklahoma, Texas
214-767-4056; TDD: 214-767-8940

Colorado, Montana, North Dakota, South Dakota, Utah, Wyoming
303-844-2024; TDD: 303-844-3439

American Samoa, Arizona, California, Guam, Hawaii, Nevada, Northern Mariana Islands
415-437-8310; TDD: 415-437-8311

Alaska, Idaho, Oregon, Washington
206-615-2290; TDD: 206-615-2296

Based on *Medicare and You,* from the Health Care Financing Administration.

HEALTH CARE FINANCING ADMINISTRATION REGIONAL OFFICES

Call these numbers for information on Medicare, Medicaid, or how to file a complaint directly with HCFA.

Connecticut, Maine, Massachusetts, New Hampshire, Rhode Island, Vermont
Boston Regional Office: 617-565-1232

New York, New Jersey, Puerto Rico, U.S. Virgin Islands
New York Regional Office: 212-264-3657

Delaware, District of Columbia, Maryland, Pennsylvania, Virginia, West Virginia
Philadelphia Regional Office: 215-861-4226

Alabama, Florida, Georgia, Kentucky, Mississippi, North Carolina, South Carolina, Tennessee
Atlanta Regional Office: 404-562-7500

Illinois, Indiana, Michigan, Minnesota, Ohio, Wisconsin
Chicago Regional Office: 312-353-7180

Iowa, Kansas, Missouri, Nebraska
Kansas City Regional Office: 816-426-2866

Arkansas, Louisiana, New Mexico, Oklahoma, Texas
Dallas Regional Office: 214-767-6401

Colorado, Montana, North Dakota, South Dakota, Utah, Wyoming
Denver Regional Office: 303-844-4024

American Samoa, Arizona, California, Guam, Hawaii, Nevada, Northern Mariana Islands
San Francisco Regional Office: 415-744-3602

Alaska, Idaho, Oregon, Washington
Seattle Regional Office: 206-615-2354

Based on *Medicare and You,* from the Health Care Financing Administration.

LONG-TERM CARE FACILITY
SELECTION PLANNER

1. FACILITY DATA

Name of facility_____

Address_____ Phone (____)_____

Contact person _____ Position _____

TYPE OF FACILITY

☐ Subacute care unit
☐ Skilled nursing facility
☐ Nursing facility (basic nursing and/or custodial care)
☐ Dementia specialized care unit
☐ Group home or community-based residential facility
☐ Assisted living
☐ Hospice

PAYER SOURCES THE FACILITY ACCEPTS OR IS APPROVED FOR

☐ Medicare
☐ Medicaid
☐ VA
☐ HMO   Name of your HMO_____
☐ Other _____

REFERENCES AND ACCREDITATION STATUS

1. _____

_____

2. _____

_____

Accredited by _____

Level of accreditation _____

2. Care and Therapy Information

TYPES OF CARE REQUIRED; CHECK ALL THAT APPLY.
MATCH THE ITEMS THAT ARE CHECKED AGAINST THE
SERVICES AVAILABLE FROM THE LONG-TERM CARE FACILITY.

NEEDED	AVAILABLE	TYPE OF CARE
☐	☐	Basic nursing care only
☐	☐	Dementia care
☐	☐	Physical therapy
☐	☐	Occupational therapy
☐	☐	Respiratory therapy
☐	☐	Speech therapy
☐	☐	Psychiatric/psychological therapy or counseling
☐	☐	IV therapy
☐	☐	Total parenteral nutrition (TPN)
☐	☐	Enteral nutrition (tube feeding)
☐	☐	Special skin care: complex burn or wound care
☐	☐	Special nutritional treatment
☐	☐	Hemodialysis or peritoneal dialysis
☐	☐	Ventilator care
☐	☐	Pain management
☐	☐	Head or spinal cord injury care
☐	☐	Cardiac rehabilitation
☐	☐	AIDS care
☐	☐	Hospice care
☐	☐	Mental illness, mental retardation, or developmental disability
☐	☐	Other _____

COMMENTS _____

_____

_____

3. PHYSICIAN INFORMATION AND VERIFICATION

Name of attending physician _____

This physician has admitting privileges in this facility.　　☐ Yes　　☐ No

If no, ask about other family practice, general practice, or geriatric specialists
with admitting privileges at this facility who are accepting new patients:

NAME   PHONE NUMBER

_____   _____

_____   _____

_____   _____

_____   _____

Facility medical director _____

4. AVAILABILITY OF BEDS

Are beds currently available for new admissions?　　☐ Yes　　☐ No

If yes, in what units (basic nursing, Medicare certified distinct part, dementia unit, etc.)?_____

_____

If no, are any vacancies anticipated?　　☐ Yes　　☐ No

If yes, by what date?_____

5. COMMENTS/QUESTIONS

_____

_____

_____

_____

6. FACILITY POLICIES

ASK FOR COPIES OF THE FOLLOWING POLICIES:

1. Admission, transfer, and discharge.
2. Residents' rights.
3. Use of physical restraints and restraint use reduction.
4. Use of psychoactive medications.
5. Emergency management of combative residents (behavioral management).
6. Fire and disaster plan.
7. Prevention and investigation of abuse, neglect, and misappropriation.
8. Room and roommate changes.
9. Bed hold policy.
10. Policy on staffing the facility on each shift.
11. Listing of services available in the facility and the charges for each.

7. STATE SURVEY INFORMATION BASED ON HCFA FORM 2567 OR OSCAR 3*

SURVEY YEAR	CITATIONS RELATED TO DEFICIENCIES IN QUALITY OF CARE, QUALITY OF LIFE, OR RESIDENTS' RIGHTS (INCLUDING INAPPROPRIATE USE OF RESTRAINTS, USE OF UNNECESSARY DRUGS, OR ABUSE/NEGLECT)
_____	_____
	_____
	_____
	_____
_____	_____
	_____
	_____
	_____
_____	_____
	_____
	_____
	_____

* On-line Survey Certification and Report 3. This report summarizes deficiencies the facility has been cited for in the past several annual surveys. If the facility has had any citations involving *substandard quality of care*, has had any enforcement actions taken such as civil money penalties imposed, or has had numerous repeat citations in the areas mentioned in the heading of the table, ask the facility for detailed information on the deficiencies cited and about the plan of correction.

8. FACILITY TOUR CHECKLIST

YES	NO	CRITERIA
		EXTERIOR AREAS
☐	☐	Grounds are clean and orderly
☐	☐	There are benches, patios, and/or walkways on the grounds
☐	☐	The building exterior appears well maintained
☐	☐	Resident outdoor activity areas are away from traffic or secured

YES	NO	CRITERIA
		INTERIOR AREAS
☐	☐	Hallways free of carts, hampers, and clutter
☐	☐	Safety handrails line the hallways
☐	☐	Dining areas clean and spacious
☐	☐	Resident rooms clean and inviting
☐	☐	Personal items and furnishings evident in resident rooms
☐	☐	Lighting adequate and free of shadows and glare
☐	☐	Rooms and hallways odor-free
☐	☐	Leisure or living areas carpeted
☐	☐	Noise levels minimal
☐	☐	Wall coverings or paint in good repair
☐	☐	Cabinetry/woodwork in good repair
☐	☐	Resident toilet rooms clean, odor-free; grab rails in place
☐	☐	Living and activity areas attractively lit and decorated
☐	☐	Therapy areas clean and well equipped
☐	☐	Nurse's station clean and located to allow good unit supervision
☐	☐	Central air conditioning
☐	☐	Private visiting areas available
☐	☐	Draft-free heating and ventilation
☐	☐	Independent living apartments available
☐	☐	Chapel/religious services available
☐	☐	Beauty/barber shop on-site
☐	☐	Sprinkler fire suppression system
☐	☐	Exit door alarms
☐	☐	Wandering resident alert system
☐	☐	Resident library or reading areas
☐	☐	Dietary services food preparation area clean and orderly
☐	☐	Tub/shower rooms clean, not used for equipment storage
☐	☐	Resident rooms, tub rooms have privacy curtains or screens
☐	☐	Residents appear well dressed and groomed
☐	☐	Privacy appears to be assured (curtains used, doors closed, etc.)
☐	☐	Staff courteous, pleasant, and professional
☐	☐	Activity/event calendar posted
☐	☐	State survey report available to residents
☐	☐	Facility has an active resident council or committee
☐	☐	Staff appear adequate in number
☐	☐	Facility performs criminal background checks on new hires
☐	☐	Physical restraints in use — Percentage of residents _____
☐	☐	Psychoactive drugs in use — Percentage of residents _____
☐	☐	Residents with skin breakdown — Percentage of residents _____
☐	☐	Incontinent residents — Percentage of residents _____